IMPROVING SUBSTANCE ABUSE TREATMENT

SAGE SOURCEBOOKS FOR THE HUMAN SERVICES SERIES

Series Editors: ARMAND LAUFFER and CHARLES GARVIN

IMPROVING SUBSTANCE ABUSE TREATMENT

An Introduction to the Evidence-Based Practice Movement

Michele J. Eliason

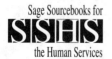

Sage Sourcebooks for
the Human Services

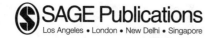

SAGE Publications
Los Angeles • London • New Delhi • Singapore

For information:

Sage Publications, Inc.
2455 Teller Road
Thousand Oaks, California 91320
E-mail: order@sagepub.com

Sage Publications Ltd.
1 Oliver's Yard
55 City Road
London EC1Y 1SP
United Kingdom

Sage Publications India Pvt. Ltd.
B 1/I 1 Mohan Cooperative
   Industrial Area
Mathura Road, New Delhi 110 044
India

Sage Publications Asia-Pacific
   Pte. Ltd.
33 Pekin Street #02-01
Far East Square
Singapore 048763

Printed in the United States of America.

Library of Congress Cataloging-in-Publication Data

Eliason, Michele J.
Improving substance abuse treatment: an introduction to the evidence-based practice movement / Michele J. Eliason.
      p. cm.—(Sage sourcebooks for the human services series)
Includes bibliographical references and index.
ISBN 978-1-4129-5130-2 (cloth: alk. paper)
ISBN 978-1-4129-5131-9 (pbk.: alk. paper)
   1. Substance abuse—Treatment. 2. Evidence-based psychiatry. I. Title.
II. Series: Sage sourcebooks for the human services series (Unnumbered)
[DNLM: 1. Substance-Related Disorders—therapy. 2. Evidence-Based Medicine. WM 270 E43i 2007]

RC564.E45 2007
362.29—dc22   2006102692

This book is printed on acid-free paper.

07   08   09   10   11   10   9   8   7   6   5   4   3   2   1

Acquisitions Editor:	Kassie Graves
Editorial Assistant:	Veronica Novak
Project Editor:	Tracy Alpern
Copy Editor:	Bill Bowers
Typesetter:	C&M Digitals (P) Ltd.
Proofreader:	Andrea Martin
Indexer:	Michael Ferreira
Cover Designer:	Candice Harman
Marketing Associate:	Thomas Mankowski

Contents

Acknowledgments

This project was initiated with funding from the Center for Substance Abuse Treatment, Practice Improvement Collaborative, Grant # 5 UDI TI12632-02. Much of this book was conceived and written while the author was still in residence at the Iowa Consortium for Substance Abuse Research and Evaluation. Consortium Director Stephan Arndt reviewed the first draft and assisted with writing the content on statistics and research designs. Anne Wallis of the University of Iowa College of Public Health contributed content to the chapter on evaluation. Kristina Barber and Kris White provided considerable support for the project as it progressed from pamphlet to book. The book was completed while the author was on sabbatical with generous support from the Institute for Health and Aging at the University of California, San Francisco. Finally, much thanks to Diana Amodia and Marty Jessup for inspiration and support.

Sage Publications would like to thank the following reviewers:

John T. Franklin, University of Detroit Mercy
Larry Ashley, University of Nevada, Las Vegas
Paul Force-Emery Mackie, Minnesota State University, Mankato
Susan L. Schoppelrey, University of Illinois at Urbana-Champaign
Steve Shoptaw, University of California, Los Angeles
Michael A. Bozarth, State University of New York at Buffalo
S. Lala Straussner, NYU School of Social Work

1

Introduction

Substance abuse and addiction is the elephant in the living room of American society. Too many of our citizens deny or ignore its presence. Abuse and addiction involving illegal drugs, alcohol and cigarettes are implicated in virtually every domestic problem our nation faces: crime; cripplers and killers like cancer, heart disease, AIDS and cirrhosis; child abuse and neglect; domestic violence; teen pregnancy; chronic welfare; the rise in learning disabled and conduct disordered children; and poor schools and disrupted classrooms. Every sector of society spends hefty sums of money shoveling up the wreckage of substance abuse and addiction. Nowhere is this more evident than in the public spending of the states. The heaviest burden of substance abuse and addiction on public spending falls on the states and programs of localities that states support. Of the two million prisoners in the United States, more than 1.8 million are in state and local institutions. States run the Medicaid programs where smoking and alcohol abuse impose heavy burdens in cancer, heart disease and chronic and debilitating respiratory ailments and where drug use is the largest cause of new AIDS cases. States fund and operate child welfare systems—social services, family courts, foster care and adoption agencies—where at least 70 percent of the cases of abuse and neglect stem from alcohol- and drug-abusing parents. The states are responsible for welfare systems that are overburdened with drug- and alcohol-abusing mothers and their children. State courts handle the lion's share of drunk driving and drug sale and possession cases. States pour billions of dollars into elementary and secondary public school systems that are more expensive to operate because of drug- and alcohol-abusing parents and teenagers. (Califano, 2001)

A s the quotation on the previous page indicates, substance abuse carries enormous costs to our states and to society in general. We are living in times of ever shrinking resources and increased costs, particularly in health care. It is more important than ever that we provide the most time- and cost-effective treatment available to the field. The substance abuse treatment field, like all other practice disciplines, has long been characterized by inconsistent, idiosyncratic practices based on one's personal experiences, folklore, intuition, particular styles of communicating, or the influence of a charismatic trainer. The gap between the treatment approaches or practices that research has shown to be effective and what is actually done in substance abuse treatment agencies is enormous. Documents such as the Institute of Medicine report "Bridging the Gap Between Practice and Research" (Lamb, Greenlick, & McCarty, 1998) and the National Treatment Plan (Center for Substance Abuse Treatment [CSAT], 2000) called for connecting practice to research, and for speeding up the process of incorporating research findings into clinical practice. Currently, it takes about 15–20 years for an evidence-based practice to move from the laboratory to the field (Balas & Boren, 2000).

Even within the field of medicine, there have been complaints that the majority of practice stems from "soft-science," opinions, clinical experience, or "tradition," rather than science. If this is true of medicine, where practitioners are highly educated professionals, would not the situation be even worse in the substance abuse treatment field? Historically, substance abuse treatment grew out of a completely different system than other health care fields, as it stemmed from a self-help, peer recovery model and grew into community-based treatment programs that were often completely independent of other health care systems (White, 1998). This system of peers helping peers arose because of public stigma and the resulting isolation from mainstream health care heightened the polarization of research versus practice that continues to influence the field today (Beutler, 2004; Morgenstern, 2000). The old tradition of learning the field via one's own recovery (an apprentice model) is slowly being replaced with a science-based educational model, but the transition has not been smooth or without growing pains. The history of the field, built on the generous spirit of those individuals in recovery themselves, must be honored at the same time that new paradigms are put into place.

This book suggests some concrete ways of bridging the gap between research findings and clinical practice by providing guidance on identifying, implementing, and maintaining evidence-based practices, clinical practice guidelines, and practice improvements. Individual agencies, regions, states, and federal agencies are all engaged in this process. In 2003, the

Center for Substance Abuse Treatment began to participate in a project already started by the Center for Substance Abuse Prevention to identify effective practices. Now an agency-wide project at the Substance Abuse and Mental Health Services Administration (SAMHSA), the National Registry for Evidence-based Practices and Programs will provide federal guidance in finding practices that have a research base. Calls for proposals from SAMHSA and the National Institutes of Health (NIH) have encouraged the use of evidence-based practices or have called for studies of adoption of new practices. Books and articles are increasingly addressing the issue of evidence-based practice (e.g., Edmundson & McCarty, 2005; Miller, Sorensen, Selzer, & Brigham, 2006; Miller, Zweben, & Johnson, 2005; Sorensen, Rawson, Guydish, & Zweben, 2003). In 2003, the Oregon state legislature passed a law requiring the use of evidence-based practices in substance abuse and mental health programs funded by the state. Clearly, the time has come to seriously discuss how best to use research findings to improve substance abuse treatment services. This book is a small step in that direction.

Challenges

The evidence-based practice movement will face a number of challenges along the way, including the lack of consensus on the terminology to use in the field. Some of these contentious terms are described as follows. A first step will be to develop a common shared language.

Addiction. While the term "addiction" is used widely among some professionals, the *Diagnostic and Statistical Manual of Mental Disorders* (DSM) uses the terms "substance abuse" and "dependence" for each substance that might be causing problems for an individual (e.g., alcohol abuse, cocaine dependence, nicotine dependence). Some authors use terms like "alcoholic" and "drug addict," whereas others believe that these terms contribute to the stigma of substance abuse. This book will use the term "substance abuse" as the generic indicator of problems related to the use of alcohol, tobacco, or other drugs. It is always a challenge to describe problems that exist along a continuum, and that are mediated by so many types of influences.

Treatment. Many people get better with the help of peer groups such as Alcoholics Anonymous and Narcotics Anonymous. Are these self-help groups, support groups, or recovery communities? Are these community-based peer groups evidence-based practices, treatment modalities, supplements to treatment, or something else? What if a 12-step group is held in a treatment program facilitated by a substance abuse counselor? What is treatment?

Person Receiving Services. Depending on the setting, the recipients of substance abuse treatment services are called patients, clients, offenders, or consumers. Do these terms relate to the kinds of interventions that these recipients are offered or to who treats them (what kind of person with what kind of training)?

Recovery. What about the term "in recovery"? Is a person in recovery for the rest of his or her life, or is there a point when he or she can be considered "recovered"? What do we really know about long-term recovery? Shouldn't more attention be paid to this as the ultimate goal of treatment? How is recovery defined?

Prevention. How do prevention and treatment efforts intersect or relate to one another? This book will focus on substance abuse treatment research and clinical practice, but clearly there needs to be more articulation of theory about the continuum of substance use and how systems of prevention and treatment can come together in more effective ways.

Evidence-Based Practice. Indeed, determining the very title of this book was a difficult decision. While many people use the term "evidence-based practice," other synonyms for this movement include research to practice initiatives, bench to bedside, treatment improvements, science to service, evidence-based treatments, research-based treatment, empirically supported treatments, and many others. For the sake of consistency, this book will stick to the term "evidence-based practice" unless referring to the work of another author who uses a different term.

Evidence-based practices are supposed to improve the outcomes of treatment. Other challenges in the field have to do with how outcomes are defined, such as the controversies about purely abstinence-based treatments versus harm reduction, and the use of legal coercion and incarceration of individuals with substance abuse problems. These controversies may affect the outcomes that are chosen as important. Some evidence-based practices may impact substance use rates, whereas others work more directly on physical health, mental health, recidivism rates, or employment. Research may help the field to understand these controversies better, but research alone does not change deeply ingrained attitudes. When stigma is involved, the best research evidence in the world makes little difference in community attitudes. Finally, the need for cultural competency means that the field no longer assumes that treatments developed for and by white men can be directly applied to women or to other underserved groups based on class, ethnicity, or sexual orientation. The field has also acknowledged that materials developed for English speakers cannot be merely translated into other languages, but must take into account the cultural differences as well. Given these challenges, the evidence-based practice movement has a rocky road ahead, but full engagement in discussions about how to implement best practices may offer some solutions to these controversies and begin the process of unifying the field.

A Working Definition of Evidence-Based Practice

Borrowing from the field of medicine, where there is a longer history of an evidence-based practice movement, an evidence-based practice is "the conscientious, explicit, and judicious use of current best evidence in making decisions about the care of individual patients" (Sackett, Rosenberg, Gray, Haynes, & Richardson, 1996, pp. 71–72). This brief definition has a few key points—"current best evidence" means that the process of evaluating the research base is ongoing. Second, it is a "judicious" practice, which means that the provider uses his or her best judgment in individual cases. In fact, the Institute of Medicine (IOM) report on evidence-based practice in health care settings outlines three components of an evidence-based practice:

> Evidence-based practice is the integration of best research evidence with clinical expertise and patient values. Best research evidence refers to clinically relevant research, often from the basic health and medical sciences, but especially from patient centered clinical research . . . clinical expertise means the ability to use clinical skills and past experience to rapidly identify each patient's unique health state and diagnosis, individual risks and benefits of potential interventions, and personal values and expectations. Patient values refers to the unique preferences, concerns, and expectations that each patient brings to a clinical encounter and that must be integrated into clinical decisions if they are to serve the patient. (IOM, 2001, p. 147)

Often the emphasis is placed predominantly on the scientific evidence, but clearly an evidence-based practice movement cannot succeed without trained and skilled clinicians who take into account their client/patient's values and unique needs. The American Psychological Association (APA) makes this even more clear in their definition of Evidence-Based Practice in Psychology (EBPP), which is defined as "the integration of the best available research with clinical expertise in the context of patient characteristics, culture, and preferences" (APA Presidential Task Force on Evidence-Based Practice, 2006, p. 273).

Overview of the Book

Chapter 2 provides a brief review of the literature on evidence-based practices or principles, including clinical practice guidelines and the latest effort to use quality improvement techniques from the corporate world in substance abuse treatment agencies (often called "practice improvements"). This book will focus on the category of evidence-based practices, but clinical guidelines and practice improvements are clearly important and will always have a place in the field.

Chapter 3 reviews the concept of evidence-based practice and suggests different ways of defining criteria for evaluating existing and new treatment methods or approaches. Examples of criteria developed by two states, Iowa and Oregon, are used as examples. The criteria used by the National Registry for Evidence-Based Practices and Programs are also reviewed. The field clearly needs to identify specific methods of defining an evidence-based practice, and these three sets of criteria provide a good starting point for this discussion on how much and what kind of evidence is needed.

Developing criteria and identifying an evidence-based practice are only the first steps. Chapter 4 focuses on adoption and implementation strategies. How does an agency get buy-in to adopt a new practice? Once an evidence-based practice has been selected, what are the steps needed to ensure that agencies and individual staff adopt and implement the practice? How can that practice be sustained and nurtured over time? We have science to inform us about what practices work (at least with certain populations under certain conditions), but we are sorely lacking in research about how to use or implement research findings in the field.

Chapter 5 outlines two kinds of outcome measures that are needed when evaluating the adoption of evidence-based practices: evaluation of the effectiveness of the treatment approach (the evidence-based practice itself) on client outcomes, and measurement of fidelity (whether staff use the approach as they were trained to use it). Both types of outcome are important. Agencies will not want to undergo costly staff training and other implementation activities unless the new practice is highly likely to improve their client outcomes. If client outcomes do not improve, it is difficult to say whether the lack of improvement is due to the practice unless the agency has fidelity data to know whether staff actually implemented the practice accurately. A relatively new way of thinking about evaluation, empowerment evaluation, is introduced as a promising practice for substance abuse treatment agencies.

Chapters 6 through 9 provide a research primer for those who need more information on the research process. These chapters will be helpful to those who must read research articles, look for clinical guidance in the research literature, write grants, or design and carry out evaluation projects. The chapters include discussion of the development of hypotheses, selecting samples, defining variables, collecting and analyzing data, and interpreting the results of research. Some discussion of protection of human subjects and dissemination of research findings is also provided. The purpose of these chapters is to demystify the research process and offer practical advice on reading research reports or articles. Chapter 10 sums up the state of the art of the evidence-based practice movement and outlines some recommendations for the future.

Because treatment effectiveness research is still in its infancy and treatment adoption and implementation studies are largely embryonic, this book does not provide a definitive list of evidence-based practices. The knowledge base in the field is constantly evolving, different agencies have different treatment needs, and clients are unique and challenging. It is highly unlikely that there will ever be one best way to treat substance abuse in all clients, or one best way to reduce wait lists, or one best way to reduce relapse rates. This book provides a broad framework for selecting practices or approaches that have some degree of research evidence and that fit the needs of an agency. It also provides suggestions for introducing new practices to an agency and for measuring their effectiveness.

Ultimately, the goal is to provide policymakers, treatment programs, and individual providers with the best possible tools to help clients achieve recovery from substance abuse, thus reducing the enormous personal pain and negative impact on the individual, family, and society. Those tools include knowledge and skills to understand research reports, to know how to evaluate the science of a practice, and to know how to implement and evaluate practices once a decision is made to adopt them in an agency. In order to achieve these goals, providers, researchers, policymakers, and the recovery and advocacy communities must come together to "co-create" knowledge. Researchers need to learn more about the practical aspects of day-to-day functioning in treatment agencies, and the politics and procedures of policymaking. Providers need to become more research-savvy and open to conducting research in their agencies. Policymakers need to look to research for answers to policy-related problems, strengthen the evidence base of policy decision making, and find ways to reward the use of evidence-based practices and research-practice collaborations in the field. This book is offered in the spirit of collaboration, which will benefit all stakeholders in the process.

2

What Are Evidence-Based Practices?

The Recovery Center, a large, full-service treatment agency, serves 12 rural counties in the Midwest. The center has 12 residential beds, but most of their clients are served in drug-free outpatient and aftercare programs. More than 70 percent of their clients have criminal justice involvement of some sort. Ellen, the new executive director, finds that the staff of 25 counselors, most of whom are middle-aged or older and in recovery themselves (the clients are largely young men), report that the agency is a 12-step facility, but on further questioning, she finds that each staff member uses an eclectic blend of practices and techniques, including three who characterize their practice as "tough love." Ellen wants to transform the agency into one that uses evidence-based practices and has one treatment philosophy, but she has no idea how to go about this.

Ellen is not alone. As there is growing pressure on treatment agencies to be accountable to their communities and funding sources, and "prove" that their services work, many administrators are grappling with the problem of bringing research into their practice arenas. This is a relatively new trend in the field. While issues of accountability, standardized outcome assessments, and professionalization of the field have been percolating for years, the Institute of Medicine (IOM) report "Bridging the Gap Between Practice and Research" (Lamb et al., 1998) stimulated a much more focused debate on the gap between research and practice than had previously existed. The report deplored the billions of dollars spent on substance abuse research that is largely ignored or unknown in the field. However, the report did not put the blame on either practitioners or researchers, but instead provided a cogent discussion of the barriers to adoption of research findings. The problems are complex, and researchers, providers, and policymakers have all contributed to a lack of communication in the field. Researchers have sometimes developed esoteric practices and procedures that are not practical to use in the field, or have not translated their findings in a user-friendly manner. The research funded by the National Institute on Drug Abuse (NIDA) and the National Institute on Alcohol Abuse and Alcoholism (NIAAA) focuses much more on animal studies, lab research, and pharmacological treatments, which are not widely used in the field, particularly in community-based treatment agencies that have little or no medical oversight. Policymakers have sometimes set requirements for treatment agencies based on public opinion rather than research, required the use of evidence-based practices without sufficient guidance or technical assistance, or contributed to laws that are contrary to research findings. And providers often do not have the skills, the support, or the time to translate research findings into practice. Their needs are pressing and immediate, and cannot wait for the 6-month follow-up data to roll in or for someone to read 50 research articles and summarize their findings. In addition, research articles or books do not help providers know how to implement new practices.

The competition for limited resources has been a major concern in the field, hindering effective collaboration. The stigma of substance abuse has led to negative attitudes among the general population, resulting in limited funding for substance abuse treatment. Consumer advocacy is less powerful in this field because of the stigma of substance abuse. People in recovery from alcohol and other drugs are less likely to want to be publicly recognized than are cancer survivors or those with other less stigmatized chronic disorders; therefore, there are fewer powerful lobbying groups advocating for substance abusers. In fact, the field's historic roots in the Alcoholics Anonymous peer support model contribute to the lack of advocacy in some ways by encouraging anonymity. Consumer advocacy in other areas of health care has resulted in a general public outcry and demand for more effective treatment services. In this field, however, the loudest voices may be from community members who do not want drug treatment programs in their neighborhoods.

Bias in Research Studies

How do we figure out what works? There are different types of treatment research methods that provide different answers. The NIDA Clinical Trials

Network was modeled after the National Cancer Institute's approach, which suggested five phases in the development of new interventions:

- Phase 1: development of hypotheses drawn from basic science research and theory.
- Phase 2: development of methods, assessment instruments, intervention manuals, identification of appropriate outcomes.
- Phase 3: the randomized clinical trial to test the intervention against treatment as usual in ideal settings (efficacy).
- Phase 4: testing the intervention with subpopulations to determine how well it generalizes.
- Phase 5: testing the intervention in real-world settings (effectiveness).

Phase 3 treatment *efficacy* studies are conducted with the most rigorous control over variables and demonstrate what works under ideal situations. Treatment *effectiveness* studies take those practices found to be efficacious and test them in more everyday clinical settings (Tucker & Roth, 2006). NIDA's Clinical Trials Network (CTN) partners academic researchers with community treatment providers to bridge the gap between efficacy and effectiveness, hopefully to infuse research into the field at a faster rate. In a way, the CTN collapses the last three phases into one. Research on the effectiveness of substance abuse treatment is relatively new.

Like all clinical sciences, research in real-world settings is difficult to accomplish. No research study is perfect, but substance abuse treatment studies are even more prone to bias than some other fields of study. Bias in research findings can result from (drawn from Leavitt, 2003):

Publication Bias: Studies with positive outcomes are more likely to be published than studies without positive findings, making some practices look better than they actually are. For example, there may be six studies that find that Treatment A is no more effective than treatment as usual, and one study that finds it to be slightly better. That one study that finds a difference is more likely to get published.

Patient/Client Selection Bias: Inclusion/exclusion criteria of many studies may screen out the very patients served most often. For example, clients with co-occurring mental health problems or criminal justice involvement are often excluded from clinical trials and other experimental research. Women of childbearing years are often excluded from drug trials. In substance abuse clinical trials, when clients with co-occurring disorders are excluded, women are disproportionately left out of research.

Confounding Factors: These are variables the researcher has no control over and are not always predictable. For example, if clients receiving a new treatment get more attention from staff, a positive outcome could be due to the increased attention rather than the treatment itself—or some combination of the two.

Randomization or Lack of Randomization: It is important that each potential client has an equal chance of getting the new intervention or treatment as usual. In some settings, such as jails and prisons, randomization may be more difficult to accomplish, or even impossible.

Blinding or Masking Procedures: Ideally, the person collecting the outcome data should not know which treatment the client received. Research team members are invested in showing that their treatment works, so may introduce unconscious bias if they are aware of group membership. Similarly, staff members may consciously or unconsciously bias research participants through staff attitudes about the practices being studied. It can be difficult in smaller community treatment programs to disguise the treatment condition.

Placebo Effects: Many clients improve if they think the treatment will be effective, whether it is or not. That is why a control or comparison group is so important. Double-blind studies, where neither the client nor the person conducting the assessment knows whether the client is getting the active ingredient, are the ideal types of studies to control for placebo effects, but this is not always possible with behavioral treatments.

Compliance and Follow-Up: If more than 20 percent of the original sample drop out before the study is completed, the findings are suspect. Since the dropout rate from substance abuse treatment as usual is close to 50 percent, many studies in this field have potentially damaging dropout rates. Follow-up is more challenging in the substance abuse treatment field than in other medical studies, because clients are more likely to have unstable housing, no jobs, and shaky familial and significant other relationships. They are often transient and drop in and out of the system.

Another form of bias may be in the practices that are chosen for study by researchers. There are two major issues related to this form of research bias—what funding sources are likely to fund and what researchers prefer to study. Researchers and treatment providers may share a common trait—they often "chase" the funding. If a request for proposals is issued, both providers and researchers might try to figure out how they can access that pot of money and devise proposals that fit funder requirements, whether or not they fit the individual's research agenda or agency strategic plan. Thus funding sources drive research agendas in the field. The research calls that come from federal funding sources—and sometimes from private foundations—are driven by politics as much as by science.

Second, researchers tend to prefer practices that are concrete, and thus easier to control. Miller, Wilbourne, and Hettema (2003) looked at the clinical trials that had been conducted on alcohol use disorder treatments and found that 20 percent were focused on pharmacotherapies, 43 percent on cognitive behavioral treatments (which are often in the form of treatment manuals), and 37 percent on all other psychosocial therapies combined. Pills and manualized treatments are the easiest to study. They may not be any more effective than more complicated treatments, but they are overrepresented in the research. There has been a bias toward "objective" treatments because studies of affective and spiritual interventions are perceived as "messy" and harder to measure. The form of science that has the most authority in the Western world privileges one kind of knowledge over all others, and thus privileges academic researchers who focus on the more observable, empirical phenomena. This means that interventions that stem from academic researchers are more likely to be studied than interventions that come from clinicians, no matter how well informed, by theory and research, these interventions are. For example, a review of the research literature on relapse prevention might suggest that Alan Marlatt's model (Marlatt & Gordon, 1985) is the most widely accepted, whereas a survey of treatment agencies would suggest that Terry Gorski's model (2000) is the most widely used. In this case, the academic researcher's work is privileged over the clinician's work in the research world, but clinicians find Gorski's model more compatible with current clinical practice, and the materials are more easily implemented (Donovan, 2003).

What Is Treatment as Usual?

The most common form of treatment in the United States is outpatient "drug-free" (nonmethadone, nonpharmacological) programs, representing about half of all treatment (Batten et al., 1993). These programs have little in common beyond not providing a place for clients to sleep. However, there has been little attempt to study what these programs actually do. What happens in the drug-free treatment program is generally referred to as "treatment as usual," and most clinical trials are multi-site studies that compare a new intervention with treatment as usual. However, some research has suggested that treatment as usual in this field is highly idiosyncratic and therefore difficult to characterize. In one study (Eliason, Arndt, & Schut, 2005), substance abuse counselors were asked what treatment philosophy characterized their practice (12-step, cognitive behavioral, motivational enhancement, therapeutic community, psychodynamic, and so on), and then rated the actual principles and methods that they used in their daily practice. There was little correspondence between the two measures. That is, many counselors said they subscribed to a 12-step philosophy, but they did not necessarily use all or even most of the12-step principles or practices. The vast majority of counselors used hybrid practices—mixtures of principles and methods from many different philosophical approaches. Some of these were contradictory, such as counselors who said they had a motivational enhancement philosophy, but used confrontation and breaking down denial frequently in their practice. A combination of 12-step and psychodynamic principles was quite common. Therefore, clinical trials and other experimental research may be comparing some new approach to a highly individualized set of hybrid techniques, making the results of such comparative research very difficult to interpret. There may be no such thing as "treatment as usual."

In spite of the relative youth of the field and the problems in conducting sound scientific research, there is a body of knowledge about the efficacy and/or effectiveness of some practices or programs. We do have some sense of what works and of some things that do not work. Are these taken into account in practice? The next section reviews some of the sound research findings and how and why they are used (or not used) in practice.

Research-Practice Gaps

Table 2.1 demonstrates just a few of the gaps between research and practice that could be addressed in order for substance abuse treatment to be more aligned with research. These represent just a sampling of the disparities between science and practice.

Bridging the Gap

Rawson, Marinelli-Casey, and Ling (2002) warned the substance abuse treatment field that maintaining the status quo by continuing to use practices not supported by research will challenge the public trust. They urged the treatment field to move toward documenting outcomes and fostering practice-research

Table 2.1   Some Examples of Research-Practice Gaps

Research shows that:	*In practice:*
Pharmacological interventions (e.g., naltrexone, buprenorphine, methadone maintenance) are effective in reducing alcohol, tobacco, and opiate craving and reduce the negative consequences of substance abuse on the individual and communities, in terms of health care costs, law enforcement, and unemployment (e.g., APA, 1995; Ball & Ross, 1991; Kiefer & Mann, 2005; Meyer & Mirin, 1979; O'Brien & McKey, 2002; O'Connor et al., 1998). Naltrexone is prescribed for less than 1% of clients who might benefit from it (Lamb et al., 1998).	Medications are rarely used because of: • Cost (insurance may not cover it and most substance abusers cannot afford it). • Lack of training/education about pharmacotherapies. • Negative attitudes about using medications to treat substance abuse. • Negative attitudes about practices that may be perceived as "harm reduction" rather than abstinence-based. • Substance abuse agencies may not have access to a health care provider with prescriptive authority.
Treatment effects are usually not seen until about 90 days into treatment—thus, treatment must be longer than that. In fact, shorter treatments are quite ineffective (e.g., Finney & Moos, 2002; NIDA, 1999).	Many residential treatments are 21 days or less in length because of: • Cost (insurance limits the days of treatment or number of sessions). • Lack of parity of physical and mental health care payments. • Treatment of substance abuse is seen as an acute episode rather than a chronic disorder.
Treatment works best when group therapy is supplemented with individual therapy (NIDA, 1999).	Most substance abuse treatment is done almost entirely in groups due to cost and time considerations and lack of adequately trained staff.
Treatment needs to address the whole person because substance abuse is a biopsychosocial and spiritual phenomenon (NIDA, 1999).	Most treatments focus on substance abuse only because of the: • Cost of holistic treatment. • Lack of training of counselors. • Lack of treatment models that are holistic rather than focused on one aspect of the person.

(Continued)

Table 2.1 (Continued)

Research shows that:	In practice:
Substance dependence is a chronic, relapsing disorder, much like diabetes or hypertension. It cannot be cured but can be managed effectively with long-term, ongoing support. Periodic relapse is to be expected (McLellan et al., 2000; Scott, Ross, & Dennis, 2004).	Dependence is treated like an acute disorder with short-term intervention in times of crisis. Relapse is seen as a failure of treatment. Abstinence is often used as the only measure of treatment success. Punishment or withholding of treatment may be used in lieu of treatment.
Randomized clinical trials have shown that several treatment approaches are efficacious: 12-step facilitation, cognitive behavioral, contingency management, motivational enhancement, relapse prevention, and so on (Hubbard et al., 1989; McCrady & Ziedonis, 2001; Miller & Wilbourne, 2002; Simpson & Brown, 1999).	Clinical trials test interventions that are usually administered in individual format, not group, and many of the types of clients served in community treatment programs are excluded from the clinical trials. Thus, there is little evidence that these approaches work in the field (effectiveness; e.g., Carroll et al., 1999). There is little research on the state of the art of substance abuse treatment—clinical trials compare some treatment approaches to "treatment as usual" but there is no consistent definition of treatment as usual.
The literature (and HIV prevention research in particular) shows that practices must be culturally specific to be effective (Castro & Garfinkle, 2003; CSAT, 1999). Dropout rates are higher for some minority clients.	Most treatment is generic—all clients get the same treatment without consideration of the role of culture (race/ethnicity, gender, sexual orientation, age, etc.).
Confrontation is not an effective practice—it results in resistance and treatment dropout (Miller & Rollnick, 2002).	Two widely used programs contain some degree of confrontation: 12-step and Therapeutic Communities. There is still a widely held belief among counselors that client denial must be "broken down" for treatment to work.
Contingency management works (Higgins et al., 1993; Higgins, 1996). Providing incentives for clean urinalyses (UAs) is effective.	There is a perception that people should not be paid for "doing the right thing." Treatment reimbursement schedules often do not allow client payment or vouchers, affecting use of this practice.

Research shows that:	In practice:
The best outcomes are achieved when drug, alcohol, and tobacco treatment occurs concurrently (Burling et al., 1991; Friend & Pagano, 2005; Joseph et al., 1990; Kalman et al., 2001; Lemon et al., 2003; Shoptaw et al., 2002).	The majority of substance abuse treatment programs do not provide tobacco treatment or even encourage clients to quit smoking while in treatment, due to prevalent myths that smoking cessation is too stressful and leads to relapse and that treatment programs will lose clients (and money) if they require tobacco treatment or do not allow clients to smoke while in treatment.
Women have better outcomes in gender-responsive programs (Grella, 1999; Grella et al., 1999; Orwin et al., 2001).	The majority of programs are "gender-neutral," meaning that they do not take into account potential gender differences in programming due to lack of training and resources to build gender-responsive programs.
Drug and alcohol educational lectures and films are ineffective (Davis et al., 1995; Miller et al., 2003).	Many treatment programs, particularly in jails and prisons, use lectures and films as part of their core curricula. Continuing education for professionals of all sorts still relies on the lecture format.

collaborations. Efforts to bridge the research-practice gap from the federal perspective have taken several forms, and most of the recommendations of the Institute of Medicine report have been initiated to some extent. The Center for Substance Abuse Treatment has been concerned with this gap between research and practice and instituted several major programs to bridge the gap:

- The **Addiction Technology Transfer Centers** (ATTCs) are charged with the dissemination of evidence-based practices to the field in forms that are tailored to different disciplines or settings. There are 14 regional ATTCs providing services to all 50 states, the District of Columbia, and Puerto Rico. Recently, the National Institute on Drug Abuse (NIDA) has partnered with ATTCs to enhance the dissemination of research findings.

- The **Practice Improvement Collaborative** (PIC) network was developed to address the adoption of evidence-based practices in the field. What are the factors that facilitate or hinder the adoption of evidence-based practices? This book started as a project of the Iowa PIC, a statewide collaboration of substance abuse treatment providers, researchers, policymakers, and consumers. (See also Edmundson & McCarty, 2005, for reports on some of the PIC projects.)

- **Strengthening Treatment Access and Retention** is a joint project between CSAT and the Robert Wood Johnson Foundation that is exploring practice improvements (described in more detail in a later section of this chapter).

- Finally, there is a SAMHSA-wide project, the **National Registry of Evidence-Based Programs and Practices** (NREPP), that is evaluating current programs for their scientific evidence. NREPP is discussed later in this chapter.

The National Institutes have also initiated efforts to bridge the gap. NIDA's **Clinical Trials Network** (CTN) was created to test substance abuse treatment interventions in multi-site, large-scale studies to bridge the gap between efficacy and effectiveness trials. The CTN required academic researchers to pair with providers in the community to develop the research agenda and to work together in conducting and interpreting research findings. At the time of this writing, the CTN had 30 studies underway or completed, nine on medications and the rest on behavioral programs or practices, such as motivational enhancement, incentives, brief strategic family therapy, and Seeking Safety (Najavits, 2002), a combined trauma and substance abuse curriculum. NIDA has also developed the **Clinical Toolbox**, which contains three treatment manuals and other documents from Project Match, a large-scale study of 12-step, cognitive behavioral, and motivational enhancement practices for the treatment of alcohol use disorders. NIDA initiated a new publication, titled *Science and Practice Perspectives,* which blends research articles with clinical feedback. This publication is available for free. NIDA is working more closely with CSAT on dissemination of research findings. The National Institute on Alcohol Abuse and Alcoholism (NIAAA) briefly had a **Researcher in Residence** program (Hilton, 2001) that paired a researcher with a provider agency. Reports of this pilot study showed benefits to both the provider organizations and the researchers who participated. These efforts at collaboration across federal agencies and cooperation in working toward greater dissemination of research findings are admirable, but their effects are not yet evident in the field.

Researchers, providers, and policymakers are governed by very different systems and performance measures. Researchers must publish in the "right" journals, generally those that cater to scientific jargon and sophisticated statistical analyses. Writing articles for practice journals or preparing treatment manuals may be frowned upon or even punished in some academic departments. Research grants are valued much more than service grants or small-scale evaluation projects. This makes it difficult for researchers to collaborate with providers and conduct field research that is mutually beneficial to the researchers (who can get data to publish out of it) and providers (who get trained in a new approach or who get outcome data to show to their funders). Both providers and researchers have to learn to accommodate each other's needs, and there needs to be external pressure or incentives of some sort on both systems to foster collaborations. The National Institutes and SAMHSA are beginning to ask for evidence of research-practice collaborations in order to qualify for some grant funding, a good first step. However, there needs to be pressure (and incentives) on academic departments to value adoption studies and applied research, and encourage practice-research collaborations as much as they value basic research. Policymakers are driven by public opinion and political climates, sometimes to the contradiction of research findings. Policymakers often must respond quickly to questions about the need for services and justify why resources need to be allocated to substance abuse treatment. Researchers are often reluctant to give the kind of strong messages/definitive answers that policymakers need to convince legislators or funding sources to provide much-needed resources. Finally, journal editors need to commit to increase the publication of articles about implementation and adoption of evidence-based practices if the field is to move ahead in infusing practice with research. In mid-2006, the *Journal of Substance Abuse Treatment* announced a new collaboration with *Counselor* magazine, whereby selected research articles printed in *JSAT* would be rewritten by the author in a format more useful to the provider audience of *Counselor* (McLellan, 2006). This is an excellent model for other journals to take—a partnering of research and clinical practice journals will certainly benefit the field.

Types of Research-Based Practices

In this section, three different types of efforts to infuse research into practice are reviewed: clinical practice guidelines or consensus statements, evidence-based practices, and practice improvements. All are useful for different purposes, and they are based on different kinds of evidence.

Clinical Practice Guidelines/Consensus Documents

Many disciplines, including the substance abuse field, have developed clinical practice guidelines as a means of making treatment more consistent from one agency to another, or from one provider to another. Clinical practice guidelines are based on current research findings and/or on consensus panels of experts in the field. They are intended to help clinicians make better decisions about treatment. Some guidelines are specific to assessment or to particular situations, such as treating the HIV-positive client, whereas some practice guidelines are broader. The purpose of clinical guidelines is the same as the purpose for evidence-based practices—to translate research into practice, increase the effectiveness of treatment, provide a framework for collecting data about treatment, ensure accountability to funding sources, and encourage some consistency in practice. One difference between clinical practice guidelines and evidence-based practices is that practice guidelines are not based on a single theoretical framework. Rather, practice guidelines are drawn from a wide variety of expert opinion and research literature, representing an eclectic collection of "things that work." Evidence-based practices are generally based on one theoretical approach and provide detailed descriptions of how to carry out the approach, whereas practice guidelines are broad general principles rather than specific procedures.

The National Institute on Drug Abuse's *Principles of Effective Drug Treatment* (1999) is an example of clinical practice guidelines for substance abuse treatment. This document outlines 13 principles of drug addiction treatment based on findings from NIDA-funded research. They include somewhat abstract concepts rather than specific procedures or techniques. The principles are:

1. No single treatment is appropriate for all individuals.

2. Treatment needs to be readily available.

3. Effective treatment attends to multiple needs of the individual, not just his or her drug use.

4. An individual's treatment and services plan must be assessed continually and modified as necessary to ensure that the plan meets the person's changing needs.

5. Remaining in treatment for an adequate period of time is critical for treatment effectiveness (a minimum of 3 months for most clients).

6. Counseling (individual and group) and other behavioral therapies are critical components of effective treatment for addiction.

7. Medications are an important element of treatment for many patients, especially when combined with counseling and other behavioral therapies.

8. Addicted or drug-abusing individuals with coexisting mental disorders should have both disorders treated in an integrated way.

9. Medical detoxification is only the first stage of addiction treatment, and by itself does little to change long-term drug use.

10. Treatment does not need to be voluntary to be effective.

11. Possible drug use during treatment must be monitored continuously.

12. Treatment programs should provide assessment for HIV/AIDS, Hepatitis B and C, tuberculosis, and other infectious diseases, and counseling to help

patients modify or change behaviors that place themselves or others at risk of infection.

13. Recovery from drug addiction can be a long-term process and frequently requires multiple episodes of treatment.

Unfortunately, this document from NIDA does not outline who selected these principles, how the principles were derived, or how scientific criteria were applied. In the future, transparency of the process is necessary to determine the credibility and the generalizability of the principles. The principles also need to be reviewed and updated in the very near future. Given the explosion of research in the field, these principles may already be out of date. However, the principles of effective treatment were a first step by NIDA to synthesize the knowledge gained through NIDA-funded research into a set of principles with clinical application.

Other practice guidelines come from professional organizations such as the American Society of Addiction Medicine (ASAM), which produces the patient placement criteria that are widely used in the substance abuse field (ASAM, 2001). ASAM also has clinical practice guidelines for pharmacological management of substance dependence. The *Diagnostic and Statistical Manual of Mental Disorders, Fourth Edition, Revised* (DSM-IV-R) criteria for substance abuse and dependence were also developed via a consensus panel, and offer guidelines for making diagnoses of substance use and mental health disorders. The American Psychiatric Association also has practice guidelines for substance abuse treatment (McCrady & Ziedonis, 2001). These types of guidelines are generally found on the Web sites or in the publication departments of professional organizations and may or may not be widely disseminated.

Consensus documents may also be published as journal articles. For example, the *Journal of Substance Abuse Treatment* published a consensus article on the effectiveness of self-help organizations. Humphreys et al. (2004), representing a SAMHSA/VA Hospital Workgroup on Substance Abuse Self-Help Organizations, reviewed the literature on the effectiveness of these groups and offered recommendations to providers and policymakers for encouraging the use of self-help groups. Join Together, a national resource center for substance abuse information, recently convened an expert panel to produce recommendations and guidelines for states in addressing substance abuse in a more comprehensive manner (Join Together, 2006).

Clinical practice guidelines generally allow great freedom in the actual implementation of the practice. For example, one NIDA guideline states that treatment needs to be readily available, but does not specify how to accomplish that. Some regions may set up treatment in schools or shopping malls; others may place treatment on job sites, in senior centers, or primary care settings. The NIDA principle about medication use does not offer help in finding ways to pay for the medications or find physicians willing to prescribe them and monitor their use.

To stay current with research, clinical practice guidelines should be reviewed and updated at least every 3 to 5 years by panels of experts from all key stakeholder groups (Lamb, Greenlick, & McCarty, 1998). Guidelines in published form are rarely implemented unless they are accompanied by other strategies, such as endorsement by professional associations, using opinion leaders for dissemination, and/or incorporating the practice guidelines into training, continuing education, and certification program requirements (Greco & Eisenberg, 1993).

Evidence-Based Practices

Evidence-based practices are generally those specific treatment approaches or procedures that have been subjected to randomized clinical trials or other experimental research designs, and have been found to be more effective than "treatment as usual." They are often developed in the form of clinical practice manuals, sets of specific procedures or techniques, or treatment modalities that are well elucidated. The manuals generally specify the length of treatment and the specific topics and approaches to be used. Many evidence-based practices are based on a specific theoretical approach, such as motivational enhancement (Rogerian theory), contingency management (operant conditioning), or cognitive behavioral methods (cognitive behavioral theory). Other evidence-based practices arose from clinical need, and later were more developed theoretically, such as the 12-step practices and therapeutic communities.

Treatment manuals were developed to improve the quality of experimental research by reducing the variability of counselor administration of a new approach, and now manuals are widely used in treatment outcome studies (Carroll, 1997). However, there are no standards for training clinicians how to use manuals (Addis, 1997; Craighead & Craighead, 1998). There is little research on the implementation process, even though manualized treatments have become the preferred form of evidence-based practices. In the field of psychology, there has been research to suggest that using treatment manuals does not necessarily improve client outcomes, and in fact, may interfere with the development of a therapeutic relationship (Miller et al., 2004).

NIDA's clinical practice manuals and the Project Match manuals are examples of clinical treatment manuals. At the time of this writing, there were three Project Match manuals (Twelve Step Facilitation Therapy, Cognitive-Behavioral Therapy, and Motivational Enhancement Therapy). NIDA also had three manuals for cocaine dependence treatment: Cognitive-Behavioral Treatment, Community Reinforcement plus Vouchers, and Individual Drug

Counseling. The Center for Substance Abuse Treatment had manuals for treatment of adolescent marijuana users. The Clinical Trials Network will likely publish other manualized treatments in the near future. For example, Lisa Najavits's (2002) *Seeking Safety* program, already published in manual form, has undergone several small-scale clinical trials with positive outcomes, and is being tested in the Clinical Trials Network with larger samples. Motivational enhancement therapy, in manual form from Project Match, has also been studied under several different conditions or with different populations in the Clinical Trials Network.

Warning: Just because a treatment approach comes in a detailed manual format does not make it an evidence-based practice. Many manuals are based only on the author's clinical experience, and there is no empirical research to support their use. Evidence-based practices come with a plethora of information about the research that went into their development and the client populations on which the practice was tested. It is vital that the research was peer-reviewed, which generally means it is published in a journal format. On the other hand, lack of empirical research to support a manual does not necessarily mean that it is "bad" or ineffective, just that it has not yet been studied.

Practice Improvements

The concept of practice improvements is drawn from the corporate world's quality improvement movement, and focuses on testing "rapid cycle" changes in procedures. The Robert Wood Johnson Foundation program, **Paths to Recovery**, and CSAT's **Strengthening Treatment Access and Retention** are grant programs that have funded a handful of agencies across the United States to explore these practice improvements. This network approaches problems from the business end of substance abuse treatment, rather than the therapeutic component. With a strong "customer" orientation, practice improvements may focus on changing procedures to reduce wait list time, or moving from scheduled appointments to making all intakes walk-ins, to rearranging program hours to do intakes or treatment groups in the evening or having a person to answer the phone around the clock rather than having an answering machine pick up calls. This approach proposes trying out a change over a short period of time, collecting data, and tweaking the procedure until the desired outcome is achieved. These short-term "experiments" are more satisfying to many providers because they can observe whether the change made a difference in a matter of days or weeks, rather than waiting for months for follow-up data from the typical research study.

Obviously, there is great value in studying the business practices of an agency. For example, providing phone reminders of appointments may decrease missed appointments and thus reduce loss of revenue and inefficient use of staff time, freeing up more resources for therapeutic activities. A useful resource is the Web site of the Network for the Improvement of Addiction Treatment (www.niatx.org), the collaboration between the Robert Wood Johnson Foundation and CSAT. This Web site includes a primer for organizational change and examples of strategies tested in several organizations to improve access and retention in treatment. For example, readers can download documents such as "5 Promising Practices: Increasing Continuation," which outlines strategies that help keep clients in treatment, such as discussing barriers to continuing in treatment with clients directly and ensuring that their needs are being met. Concrete examples of how programs do this are provided. (For example, one residential program instituted monthly focus groups, and another had clients complete session rating scales after each appointment.) These practices do not meet the criteria for an evidence-based practice as discussed in Chapter 3, but could be studied experimentally in the future.

Some Challenges to the Evidence-Based Practice Movement

Recently, the high value placed on randomized clinical trials as the "best" evidence in several fields, including substance abuse, has been challenged. Victora, Habicht, and Bryce (2004) asked the field of public health to reconsider the heavy reliance on randomized clinical trials (RCTs) as the absolute form of evidence. Their arguments make good sense for the substance abuse treatment field as well. Both public health and substance abuse treatment are areas where randomized clinical trials might not always be feasible, are not always ethical, and/or do not adequately answer the research question. In a field as complex as human behavior and addiction, it is unlikely that any study can adequately control all possible explanations for the outcomes. Green (2006) noted that "most of the evidence is not very practice-based" (p. 406) and he proposes "systems science": Instead of rigidly controlling variables, as is done in clinical trials, Green recommends conducting deep analysis of all the messy everyday influences on behavior. Even if we accept the RCT as one of the best forms of evidence, the RCTs in the substance abuse treatment field have been almost entirely fairly brief individual therapies delivered by highly educated, highly trained professionals using manuals, and they have not used a chronic care model of substance abuse (Miller, 2006). In reality, most substance abuse treatment is group-oriented, and delivered over a longer period of time by a paraprofessional staff without manuals. The gap between the research and actual practice is much too large to bridge simply from RCT to community-based treatment in any easy manner.

Another issue is the accuracy and scientific rigor of journal articles. Leavitt (2003) noted that at least half of all articles in research-oriented journals contain significant errors that could impact the validity of the findings. Sometimes only researchers sophisticated in statistics and research design can identify these errors. More partnerships between applied researchers and statisticians may be needed to ensure the accuracy of the research base. If the average researcher makes these errors, how could policymakers or providers without a research background be expected to identify which studies have methodological flaws?

Scott Miller and colleagues have also been critical of the evidence-based practice movement and have suggested instead the need for "practice-based evidence." These authors note the explosion of new therapies in recent years, while research shows that most of them result in fairly equivalent outcomes (Lambert, 1992). In their search for "what works" in therapy, Hubble, Duncan, and Miller (1999) pointed to four main factors that contribute to client change:

1. Extratherapeutic influences (life circumstances of the client that occur outside of the treatment realm) contribute to 40 percent of change.

2. Relationships between client and therapist account for 30 percent.

3. Placebo, hope, and expectations contribute 15 percent of change efforts.

4. Specific treatment models or techniques account for 15 percent.

Hubble et al. (1999) proposed that providers mindfully address the extratherapeutic factors in treatment by talking about them and encouraging development of resources from the client's own world. The selected therapy approach should be compatible with the client's own theory of change and style, and therapists should check in frequently to ensure that clients are benefiting from the therapy. This body of work is quite compatible with the practice improvement movement of being "customer oriented" and searching for ways to improve services or outcomes in addition to focusing on specific therapeutic approaches. For example, monitoring of client satisfaction and progress at the end of every session provides immediate feedback to counselors about client perceptions, and the data can be used to make changes in therapeutic approach or referral in the short term. This is also compatible with the IOM definition of evidence-based practice, as it focuses on not only the specific therapeutic approach but also the client's needs and values and the therapeutic relationship.

There is a growing body of knowledge about the value of a positive counselor-client relationship (Barber et al., 1999; Bell, Montoya, & Atkinson, 1997; Kasarabada, Hser, Boles, & Huang, 2002), and if Hubble et al. (1999) are correct, this relationship is roughly twice as important as the type of therapeutic approach used. The search for evidence-based practices must not ignore the role of therapeutic relationship. Some evidence-based practices may be effective because the training or specific techniques help counselors to be better listeners or attend to certain aspects of the client's needs.

Finally, there may be a need for different kinds of evidence for different aspects of the system. Eisenberg (in Havighurst, Hutt, McNeil, & Miller, 2001) suggested that there are three levels within health care systems: the clinical level, or client care decisions; health care systems, or treatment philosophies and service delivery models; and the public policy level, or the legal, ethical, and fiscal issues, such as access to treatment or achieving parity. Randomized clinical trials may be useful in studying a specific practice, such as the therapeutic community, but not so helpful in exploring issues of parity or access to treatment strategies.

Conclusions

Let us return to the case that opened this chapter. Executive Director Ellen might be frustrated by the state of the art of the evidence-based practice movement at this point in time. She might carefully review the model programs listed on the NREPP Web site and fail to find any that are appropriate for her agency. Ellen might like to offer buprenorphine treatment, but she has no medical staff available. She may purchase the ASAM patient placement guidelines, only to find that her region does not have even half of the treatment options outlined in the document. Placement decisions are not difficult when there are only one or two choices for treatment. She may be drawn to the practice improvement or practice-based evidence models, because these are the most appealing in clinical settings and have the greatest short-term impact.

In conclusion, there are many ways to improve substance abuse treatment using research findings. While this book focuses on the evidence-based practice movement, clinical practice guidelines and practice improvements will always be helpful adjuncts to treatment improvement efforts. It is also important to listen to the critics of evidence-based practices to keep a perspective on the limitations of the approach. Keep in mind that the Institute of Medicine (2001) report defined evidence-based practice as a combination of scientifically supported treatments with clinical expertise and client values and needs. It is sometimes easy to lose sight of the complexity of treatment for substance abuse and focus too narrowly on the specific techniques or practices.

3

Determining What Is Evidence-Based

What Is "Evidence"?

Although "evidence-based practice" has become a buzzword in the last few years, there is still no consensus on what exactly constitutes evidence. What kind of evidence is needed? How much evidence? Is one very large-scale clinical trial enough? Are five experimental studies with positive outcomes enough? Leavitt (2003) suggested a "hierarchy of evidence," ranking types of research reports from the most valuable and scientifically rigorous to the least useful. Figure 3.1 shows the ranking from the most rigorous at the top of the pyramid to the least scientifically rigorous at the bottom.

Systematic Reviews and Meta-Analysis of Randomized Clinical Trials (RCTs). Once several RCTs are available, the data from them can be pooled and a sophisticated analysis can be done to determine whether the practice has no, small, medium, or large effects on outcome measures (referred to as effect size). Meta-analysis uses the individual studies as the unit of analysis rather than pooling all the subjects. There are only a few practices in the substance abuse treatment literature that have a sufficient number of RCTs to even consider meta-analysis. For example, there are two meta-analyses available concerning outcomes of naltrexone (Kranzler & van Kirk, 2001; Streeton & Whelan, 2001), but fewer for behavioral interventions. Systematic reviews are more feasible. In this approach, all the research literature on a particular practice is gathered and examined for the "big picture." Are the findings consistent across a number of studies? Examples of systematic reviews include Miller, Sorensen, Selzer, and Brigham's (2006) review of the literature on

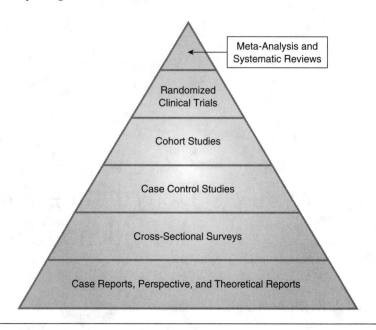

Figure 3.1   The Hierarchy of Scientific Evidence

dissemination of evidence-based practices, and Miller and Wilbourne's (2002) review of treatments for alcohol use disorders. Both systematic reviews and meta-analysis can suffer from combining studies with different client populations, different treatment settings, and different outcome measures. Sometimes it is hard to gather all the relevant literature across the multiple sources of information available, biasing the study by relying only on the studies published in major journals that are readily available.

Randomized Clinical Trials (RCTs). In this type of experimental study, clinical treatment agencies are selected as the sites rather than controlled lab settings, and clients are carefully selected according to inclusion and exclusion criteria. Clients are randomly assigned to treatment condition(s) or treatment as usual, and followed for a minimum of 6 months after treatment completion. Examples of RCT reports include the Linehan et al. (2002) study that compared dialectical behavior therapy and 12-step treatment for opioid-dependent women with borderline personality disorder, and the Project Match Research Group (1998) that compared 12-step facilitation, motivational enhancement therapy, and cognitive behavioral skills training treatment for clients with alcohol use disorders.

Cohort Studies (also called prospective, incidence, or follow-up studies). This is the most common type of research study and involves an experimental group and a control or comparison group who are followed before, during, and after treatment. However, the participants might not be randomly assigned and are drawn from convenience samples (such as people already in treatment rather than recruited specifically for the study). Examples of cohort studies include Knight, Simpson, and Hiller's (1999) 3-year follow-up study of men enrolled in therapeutic community treatment in prison and aftercare in the community. (Researchers cannot randomly assign some people to prison, as much as they might like to!)

Case-Control Studies. In this design, clients are selected on the basis of some outcome, and then the researcher looks backward in time to compare the clients. For example, a study might compare clients who dropped out of treatment to those who stayed for the duration of the treatment, looking at their intake assessments for clues about why some dropped out. However, depending on records or recall of information from the past can result in much bias. Eliason and Amodia (2006) looked at the records of more than 100 clients who were admitted to a residential program for clients with co-occurring disorders to get some ideas about who was likely to be successful in such a program.

Cross-Sectional Surveys (also called prevalence or epidemiological studies). This type of research looks at a particular group of clients at one point in time. For example, household studies of alcohol and drug use give a snapshot view of who is using what substance at one point in time. These studies might demonstrate associations, but cannot examine cause-and-effect relationships. Studies that have examined the prevalence of smoking among clients in drug treatment are examples of cross-sectional research (e.g., Richter, Ahluwalia, Mosier, Nazir, & Ahluwalia, 2002).

Case Reports. These are published studies of new approaches, unusual or unexpected events, or specific agency changes. For example, reports of adverse effects of new pharmacological treatments, or reports about new substances of abuse, or examples of how a program implemented an evidence-based practice are useful, but do not constitute strong evidence. These are useful for topics that we know little about, but do not constitute solid evidence of anything. For example, the *Journal of the American Medical Association* published a case study of a 35-year-old physician with an opioid dependence, useful for teaching purposes, but not helpful as a source of "evidence" (Knight, 2004).

Perspective or Theoretical Reports. These articles present personal opinions and clinical experiences, propose new theoretical frameworks to be tested, or offer commentary about some controversy in the field. They do not offer any scientific evidence, but may be helpful in identifying prevalent attitudes or viewpoints in the field or in identifying barriers to adoption of new practices. As an example, Rawson, Marinelli-Casey, and Ling (2002) raised a challenge to the field to develop practice and research collaborations.

Even when scientific rigor is demonstrated and the practice works in several controlled studies, will it be effective in the real world? A practice can have excellent research qualities—it can be extensively tested with randomized clinical trials, have a detailed treatment manual, and perform well with a variety of clients in controlled research studies, but still not meet practical considerations that determine its applicability to the field. For example, if it is costly to train staff, if the manuals are expensive or complicated, or if insurance or other forms of payment do not cover the cost of the treatment, the practice is not likely to be used in the field. Scientific merit is necessary, but not sufficient, as a measure of an evidence-based practice. The next section reviews three examples of attempts to identify criteria for an evidence-based practice.

Three Efforts to Develop Criteria for Evidence-Based Practices

In this section, three different efforts to define evidence-based practices—two of them at the state level, and one federal agency's response—are described. Each of these three groups took a different approach to the process and developed definitions and criteria that are similar in many ways, but dramatically different in others. At the end of this chapter, some concrete suggestions are proposed for local or state agencies or groups who want to begin the process of identifying evidence-based practices.

The Iowa Experience

In 1999, Iowa was granted a Practice Improvement Collaborative (PIC) grant to develop an infrastructure for enhancing communication among providers, policymakers, and researchers. There was already a structure in place to build upon. The Iowa Consortium for Substance Abuse Research and Evaluation was formed in 1991 as a collaboration of the state providers association, researchers from four state universities, and state-level policymakers in public health, corrections, and drug control policy. Until the late 1990s, the Consortium was involved primarily with assisting the state in evaluation projects and collecting needs assessment data, and had limited contact with the provider community. The PIC grant allowed for an expansion of the network. In 2002, the Single State Authority director asked the PIC for assistance in infusing community-based treatment agencies with evidence-based practices. The eventual goal was to tie funding to demonstration of evidence-based practice. The first step in this project was to develop a set of criteria to evaluate new and existing practices; therefore, a committee of policymakers, providers, and researchers was convened to carry out this task. The resulting criteria combined demonstration of research evidence with practical considerations. Each of the 13 criteria is outlined below, along with a rationale for its inclusion and its limitations as a criterion measure. These criteria are an attempt to operationalize evidence-based practice for the state and are a work in progress.

The 13 Iowa Criteria

1. At least one randomized clinical trial has shown this practice to be effective.

Clinical trials are considered among the best research methods to test new or existing practices. They can be the most scientifically rigorous of the types of studies done on treatment effectiveness. In a randomized clinical trial, each research participant has an equal chance of being assigned to the experimental treatment or the comparison or control group, which is typically treatment as usual. However, there are often strict inclusion and exclusion criteria to qualify for a clinical trial. The committee specified what was meant by a clinical trial, and the research had to include the following scientific elements:

- The results of the clinical trial have appeared in a refereed professional publication or journal.
- The trial adequately addressed missing data in the analyses, including subject attrition.
- The manner in which data were collected was adequate, including multiple outcome measures, if appropriate, and an adequate follow-up period.
- The relevance and quality of the outcome measures must be specified, including reliability and validity.
- The data analysis is appropriate and technically adequate.
- The trial addressed plausible threats to validity.
- The outcomes were assessed in a blinded fashion (the person collecting outcome data did not know the group assignment of the client).

- The data were obtained prospectively (in real time, not in a retrospective review).
- There was a clear presentation of inclusion and exclusion criteria for the study (who they accepted and who they did not).
- The sample size was large enough to offer reasonable statistical power and a stable estimate of the effect size.
- The statistical methods were described clearly and in sufficient detail.
- The diagnostic methods were appropriate and adequate (they adequately measured drug abuse or dependence or mental health diagnoses).

Clearly this complicated criterion focuses on the scientific merit of the study and would require a statistician or very sophisticated quantitative researcher to be able to completely evaluate whether the study met these criteria. However, even if a research study meets all these qualifications, there can still be problems in translating the research finding to a clinical setting. Clinical trials often do not mimic real life. They may exclude the very types of clients who make up most of the treatment population (such as clients with co-occurring disorders or criminal justice involvement), and they often pay clients to participate. Incentives alone may affect treatment outcomes, regardless of the intervention. If positive outcomes are reported, are they due to the treatment, the incentives, or some inseparable combination of the two? Clinical trials generally include extensive ongoing staff training and supervision, they have detailed treatment manuals, and they are often conducted in larger agencies with research experience. Clinical trials are usually designed to test treatment efficacy—does the treatment work under ideal circumstances—and they often do not attend to practicality issues (treatment effectiveness). Treatment effectiveness studies are relatively rare, especially in the substance abuse treatment field. There are not very many clinical trials that meet the Iowa criteria in the research literature because these studies are very expensive and time-consuming. In the substance abuse treatment field, where treatment dropout rates are very high, the studies often end up with an insufficient number of participants to draw any solid conclusions.

2. The practice has demonstrated effectiveness in several replicated research studies using different samples, at least one of which is comparable to the treatment population of our region or agency.

Because of the expense and difficulty involved in conducting clinical trials, other scientific research methods must be considered so that we do not overlook practices or procedures with considerable evidence of their usefulness. If several studies with different samples and in different regions report positive outcomes—even if they do not have random assignment of subjects into groups—the approach is certainly promising. However, if an agency is going to go to the considerable expense of adopting a new practice, agency officials want to be reasonably sure that the practice will work with their clients. Hence, the Iowa committee added the clause about comparability to the treatment population under question. It may be difficult to find studies with similar samples to the population served in a particular agency. In the Midwest, most treatment agencies treat rural clients with methamphetamine problems—are they comparable to urban cocaine users or even urban meth users? Studies of methamphetamine use in California show quite different client profiles of meth users than studies of meth use in Nebraska. Can the research on what works for urban gay men meth users generalize to treatment for poor white women meth users in prison in Iowa? How do we know what differences matter and which ones do not? Twelve-step programs work reasonably well for many men and women, regardless of geographical region. Would the same thing be true of motivational interviewing, the Matrix Model of stimulant abuse, or *Seeking Safety,* a post-traumatic stress disorder (PTSD) and substance abuse curriculum? Until there are studies with many different kinds of samples in different kinds of settings, it is difficult to determine if the practice is generalizable.

3. The practice either targets behaviors or shows good effect on behaviors that are generally accepted outcomes.

If the practice does not target the outcome measures collected by the agency, it will not appear to be effective, even if clients improve in other ways. The practice should target outcomes that are important to the agency. For example, a criminal justice agency may wish to impact recidivism rates. If abstinence is the major outcome measure for your agency, as it is in many places, the practice must improve abstinence rates. Some agencies may focus more on staff outcomes than on client outcomes. Are staff well trained to use the new practice, and do they use it consistently over time? Does each staff member deliver the intervention in the same way? Fidelity of treatment intervention could be an outcome measure for the implementation of a new practice. Ultimately, however, funding sources want client outcome data, not staff outcomes.

Substance abuse is a chronic relapsing disorder, so outcomes should be as broad as possible. No practice will "cure" substance abuse. However, outcome measures are often politically motivated, so they are not always consistent with research. Most states and the federal agencies that deal with substance abuse treatment are grappling with the best ways to measure outcomes in the field. At this point, there are no universally accepted outcome measures in the field.

4. The practice can logistically be applied in our region, in rural and low-population-density areas.

Some practices are highly specific, such as methadone maintenance for clients dependent on heroin. There may be an insufficient number of heroin users in a rural community to sustain the program. Gender-specific treatment approaches appear to work, but if there are only a few women at any given time in an agency's residential program, a separate program may not be feasible. Medications may be highly effective in reducing craving for alcohol or other drugs, but if the agency has no medical oversight, or its payers will not cover medications, a pharmacological intervention is not feasible. Staff must be able to deal with all clients who come in the door with their existing resources. Few treatment effectiveness studies have been conducted in rural or frontier communities, so it may be difficult to find appropriate practices. In rural areas, treatment providers are usually generalists because specialization is not feasible. This criterion is specific to a rural state like Iowa, and would obviously not be of use to regions with large cities or high population densities.

5. The practice is feasible: It can be used in group format, is attractive to third-party payers, is of low cost, and training is available.

Practices with the highest-quality research support will not be implemented if they do not meet practical considerations. Naltrexone, for example, is quite effective in reducing alcohol craving, and there is a substantial and rigorous scientific basis for its use (Kiefer & Mann, 2005). However, if the treatment agency has no physician, or a capitated payment system, it cannot use it. Another practice, such as dialectical behavior therapy, may be very promising with certain client populations, such as those with borderline personality disorder, but requires a very high level of training or education, which is costly. On the other hand, if too much weight is put on the practical aspects, the scientific merit may be downplayed and the field will continue to use practices that are not the best available, just because they are inexpensive and easy to administer. Creative ways to finance training or purchase new materials must be sought. On reflection, this criterion combines too many disparate elements, and each one should be considered separately. Any one of these barriers may result in rejecting a practice as not feasible.

6. The practice is manualized or sufficiently operationalized for staff use. Its key components are clearly laid out.

An evidence-based practice must contain enough detail so that all staff can use the practice in the same way. Treatment manuals enhance fidelity. If staff members are not consistent in their use of a practice, the practice cannot be accurately evaluated. Treatment manuals by nature are rigid and highly specific and may inhibit counselor creativity or use of intuition. In addition, they may not lend themselves well to a particular setting. For example, if a driving under the influence (DUI) program manual has 10 one-hour sessions, but violators in one region are mandated to attend 8 hours of treatment, which 2 hours are omitted? Another issue has to do with how much adapting or modifying of a manual one can do before it is no longer an evidence-based practice. There are regional differences in language, so if the counselor uses the local "slang" or dialect, instead of the words used in the manual, is it still the same practice? Finally, research has shown that one of the most important aspects of treatment is counselor warmth and empathy (Miller & Rollnick, 2002). Are warmth and empathy reduced when counselors rigidly follow a treatment manual?

7. The practice is well accepted by providers and clients.

Buy-in by staff and treatment motivation of clients are enhanced when they accept the practice. Methadone clinics have had to fight battles in many communities because of the greater stigma attached to addiction replacement types of treatment. This stigma is found in local communities as well as among some substance abuse treatment professionals. Some communities have refused to allow halfway houses in certain neighborhoods. Similarly, substance abuse counselors may have deeply ingrained beliefs about what works and what does not work in treatment, and may be resistant to a new practice no matter how much scientific evidence there is to support it. A good example is the resistance to contingency management. Paying people for clean urine samples is a quite effective treatment, but contrary to the core beliefs of many substance abuse counselors.

Acceptability can be derived from folklore, dogmatic beliefs, or other factors totally unrelated to the effectiveness of a practice. Providers and clients alike tend to prefer the old familiar practices and are resistant to change. Focusing too much on acceptability maintains the status quo, but ignoring acceptability can result in outright rejection of the practice or can undermine change efforts.

8. The practice is based on a clear and well-articulated theory.

Theory-driven practice is preferred to eclectic, atheoretical approaches because theories are usually testable. The scientific method begins with generating hypotheses from theories, and then testing those hypotheses. However, treatment effectiveness may be related to highly specific behaviors or skills within a theory. That is, the theory may lack validity, but some of its components may still work. Substance abuse is a complex biopsychosocial phenomenon that may defy the development of any unified grand theory. Most treatment approaches or practices today are somewhat overlapping and are not theoretically distinct (Eliason, Arndt, & Schut, 2006). Twelve-step programs use many components of a cognitive behavioral intervention, and motivational interviewing is client-centered, but also draws on cognitive theory. The latest innovation in the field, using principles of quality improvement drawn from the business world, proposes a more atheoretical, empirical approach. Experts in this field recommend "rapid cycle" changes—making a small change in the way the agency is run and noting the short-term effects. If there are no effects in a short period of time, abandon the approach and try something else. Can these practice improvements be considered evidence-based practices if they are not grounded in theory? Much of what is done in the field is based more on common sense and needs assessment data than on theory.

9. The practice has associated methods of ensuring fidelity.

Fidelity (consistent delivery of the treatment over time) is a key component in evaluating the effectiveness of a treatment. If staff members alter a practice in ways that have not been studied empirically, the practice is no longer evidence-based. Research on fidelity is even newer than treatment effectiveness research. There are few well-established methods of measuring fidelity. The best methods (e.g., direct observation by a third party) may be cost-prohibitive, whereas the least expensive methods (self-report measures such as checklists) may not be very accurate. In Iowa, motivational interviewing training was implemented in 2003. A condition of receiving free training was that the staff members send in two audiotapes of sessions with clients for fidelity checks and feedback about their use of the procedure. The vast majority of trainees failed to return their audiotapes, even when provided with tape recorders and given frequent reminders to make their tapes.

10. The practice can be evaluated.

Evaluation, or the measurement of behavioral outcomes (staff and client), is an essential part of research on treatment effectiveness. It is also a form of accountability to a funding source or a community. Just because a program or practice is evidence-based does not mean that it will necessarily work for the clients at a particular agency. The outcomes must match the treatment objectives. For example, if job training is a major part of the treatment approach—because unemployment is a major relapse risk factor—then change in employment status must be one of the outcome measures. Another issue is related to the timing of the evaluation. If outcome measures are collected at the time of treatment completion, the results are much different than if outcome measures are collected 6 months after treatment completion. Each agency or region must determine when to evaluate as well as how to evaluate. When evaluating the implementation of an evidence-based practice, measuring staff outcomes may be as important as measuring client outcomes. See Chapter 5 on evaluation for some guidelines in developing an evaluation plan.

11. The practice shows good retention rates for clients.

High dropout rates adversely affect outcomes, thus one common outcome measure in research studies is the percentage of clients who receive the new practice who complete treatment compared to those in the treatment-as-usual condition. If a practice requires a very high level of cognitive functioning, or benefits only a specific segment of the population, overall dropout rates may be high, but specific subgroups may have much lower dropout rates. Sometimes clients can be dropped from a program because of low attendance; however, frequent attendance may be difficult for those who are elderly, have no transportation, or who have inflexible jobs. Good screening procedures may be needed to identify the clients who will really benefit from the practice. Just throwing all clients into the same pot may be the problem, rather than the practice itself. For example, in one study, clients with no mental health diagnoses had much higher dropout rates than clients with severe mental illness—the program was for clients with co-occurring disorders, so the clients with no mental health diagnosis were probably inappropriately placed (Eliason & Amodia, 2006). Alternatively, staff attitudes may be a problem. If staff have not committed to the practice, they may send mixed messages to clients, who in turn become suspicious of the practice.

12. The practice addresses cultural diversity and different populations.

Agencies often cannot afford to offer many highly specific approaches. They need practices with wide applicability, or that have modifications or adaptations for different populations. For example, only larger agencies tend to have special programs for the older adult (Schutte, Nichols, Brennan, & Moos, 2003). Some agencies are culturally specific and must determine whether an evidence-based practice fits the cultural norms of the group that they serve. Many Native American programs use a Native American–specific approach such as the Red Road to Recovery or medicine wheels, which may not be relevant to other racial or ethnic groups. Some faith-based programs are appropriate for clients with compatible religious beliefs, but inappropriate for other clients. Clients are extremely diverse, and it may be difficult to find practices that are appropriate for all. Adolescents and elderly clients have very different needs; women with children have different needs than single men.

Should agencies specialize in different kinds of clients? This may not be feasible in rural areas. Small, generic agencies need practices that can be widely used. Thus far, the discussion of evidence-based practices nationwide has not adequately addressed issues of diversity. This may be one of the most significant shortcomings of the movement at this point in time. It is highly unlikely that any one treatment approach or technique will be effective for all clients.

13. The practice can be used by staff with a wide diversity of backgrounds and training.

Substance abuse professionals range from people with no higher education at all to people with PhDs or MDs. They also vary widely in the type and amount of training they have received, and whether they are in recovery themselves. Although counselor competencies have been identified (TAP 21, CSAT 1998), they are not consistently applied in the field. Some of the best practices require a great deal of training, and therefore, will rarely be adopted. Professionalization of the field may be necessary before more complex treatment approaches will be consistently used in the field. A certain level of formal education with coursework on basic counseling competencies as well as specific evidence-based practices is needed. Clinical supervision may be another key element in implementing a new practice. If only line staff were trained, but not their supervisors, the supervisors may be unable to facilitate the adoption of the practice and give the type of feedback that is required to really learn a new practice.

Conclusion and Application

In conclusion, there are problems with each of the Iowa criteria, and they are not clear-cut and precise. Individual states or regions may want to modify these criteria for their own use. It is important that the criteria address all the major concerns of a particular agency or region, or they are merely an intellectual exercise.

The Evidence-Based Practice (EBP) Committee in Iowa used the 13 criteria to identify a practice for a pilot implementation project. Motivational Interviewing (MI) met the majority of the criteria with solid scientific evidence, wide acceptability, and availability of training. Table 3.1 shows how MI fits the Iowa criteria.

The Oregon Mandate

Oregon has a unique experience in the implementation of evidence-based practices. In 2003, the state legislature introduced and passed Senate Bill 267

Table 3.1   Applying the Iowa Criteria to Motivational Interviewing

Criteria	Motivational Interviewing
Randomized clinical trials	Yes
Several replicated studies with different populations	Yes
Targets accepted outcomes	Yes—retention in treatment, reduction in drug or alcohol use
Logistically feasible	Yes—can be used in a variety of settings, appropriate for rural settings
Feasible in groups and to payers, low cost, training available	In general, yes. Training cost is somewhat high but can be used in groups and training is available.
Manualized or operationalized	Yes, good training and clinical materials are available.
Well accepted	Yes
Based on theory	Yes
Has fidelity measures	Yes, although difficult to get counselors to do them and is time consuming and costly.
Can be evaluated	Yes
Affects retention rates	Yes
Addresses cultural diversity	To some extent—has been used with many different populations successfully.
Can be used by staff with wide diversity of backgrounds	Yes, to some extent. The general skills can be taught fairly easily, whereas the overall approach is somewhat more complex and requires a fair amount of study and lots of practice to master it.

(see Appendix A for a copy of the bill). This bill mandated five state agencies, including the substance abuse, mental health, and criminal justice systems, to demonstrate the use of evidence-based practices or lose their funding. The time frame for implementation mandated that by 2005, agencies must show that 25 percent of their state funds were used to support evidence-based practices. By 2007, the percent must increase to 50 percent, and by the final phase, in 2009, 75 percent of funds must be devoted to evidence-based practices.

In response to the legislation, the state Office of Mental Health and Addiction Services (OMHAS) drafted a six-tier definition of evidence-based practice, after recognizing that substance abuse treatment approaches fall along a continuum of effectiveness. The six tiers of evidence include:

• *Level I:* The practice is supported by scientifically sound experimental studies that consistently show positive outcomes, and those positive outcomes have been identified in both scientifically controlled and real-world settings.

• *Level II:* The practice is supported by experimental studies that consistently show positive outcomes. These positive outcomes have been demonstrated in scientifically controlled or routine care settings, but not both.

• *Level III:* A practice which originally met Level I or II criteria, but has been modified for or applied to a different population than the original research, or a practice that is difficult to study in typical experimental research.

• *Level IV:* A practice that is intended to fill a gap in the system; a promising procedure that is currently undergoing testing.

• *Level V:* A practice that is not based on research, or the existing research is not replicable. A practice based on clinical opinion or non-experimental research.

• *Level VI:* A practice that has several experimental studies that demonstrates poor outcomes or causes harm.

Levels I to III are deemed "evidence-based practices" for the purposes of the law, although the Oregon drug and alcohol program administration recognize that there will always be a need for the Level IV practices as well. The onus will be on individual providers to demonstrate that they are using Level I, II, or III practices. Table 3.2 shows how these six tiers of evidence compare on six important dimensions: transparency, research, standardization, replication, presence of a fidelity scale, and meaningful outcomes. These terms are defined below.

The criteria and definitions were widely distributed in the field for comment, and are now in the early process of implementation. Oregon has used a three-step process to meet the mandate. The three steps are:

1. Develop operational definitions of EBP and present them for stakeholder review and discussion (see definitions in Table 3.2).

2. Establish an internal steering committee to review policy issues. This committee includes an EBP Unit that spearheads implementation and provides technical assistance to the field. The technical assistance is on the adoption of specific EBPs and is given at no or low cost.

Table 3.2 Oregon Criteria for Evidence-Based Practice

Level	Transparency	Research	Standardization	Replication	Fidelity	Outcomes
I	Yes	≥ 3 studies in peer-reviewed journals, one of which is an RCT	Yes	Yes	Yes	Yes
II	Yes	≥ 3 studies in peer-reviewed journals at least quasi-experimental	Yes	Yes	In development or No	Yes
III	Yes	≥ 3 studies in peer-reviewed journals, not rigorously controlled	Yes	No	No	Yes
IV	Yes	0–2 studies	No	No	No	Maybe
V	No	None	No	No	No	No
VI	Yes	Yes	Yes	Yes	No	No

Explanation of terms in the table:

- Transparency: both the criteria (how to find evidence, what qualifies as evidence) and the process (who reviews the evidence) should be open to observation by the public.
- Research: the accumulated scientific evidence is based on randomized clinical trials (RCTs), quasi-experimental studies, and in some cases, less rigorously controlled studies. Research should be published in appropriate peer-reviewed journals and available for review. Limited exceptions may be granted for nonpublished research, if it is of sufficient quality, documented, and available for review.
- Standardization: an intervention must be standardized in some way so that it can be replicated elsewhere by others. Standardization typically involves a manual or book that clearly defines the practice and some measures to assess if the intervention is being accurately practiced.
- Replication: more than one study finds similar positive effects when clients/consumers receive the service.
- Fidelity Scale: a fidelity measurement is used to verify that an intervention is being implemented in a manner consistent with the treatment model or the research that produced the practice.
- Meaningful outcomes: effectiveness interventions must show that they can help clients/consumers to achieve important goals or outcomes related to impairments and/or risk factors.

3. Develop policies and procedures for identifying, evaluating, approving, and listing EBPs. This includes working with accreditation bodies to ensure that they focus more closely on EBP theory and practice, conducting fidelity reviews of agencies, and updating management information systems to accommodate the new systems.

In Fiscal Year 2005, the OMHAS surveyed providers and estimated that 56 percent of public funds was being spent to support EBPs in drug and alcohol treatment and prevention programs. At the time of this writing, the state was working to define the requirements for providers as well as develop a system of incentives for adoption of EBPs, and changing fee structures to increase reimbursement rates for EBPs and reduce payment for non-EBP services. The state was providing a list of approved evidence-based practices for agencies to consider (see Table 3.3). It will be critical for the rest of the nation to observe how Oregon's system works.

The Federal Response: National Registry of Evidence-Based Programs and Practices (NREPP)

In 1998, the Substance Abuse and Mental Health Services Administration (SAMHSA) developed a procedure for evaluating individual practices and programs. SAMHSA officials use panels of experts to evaluate nominated practices and programs using both methodological and appropriateness criteria. The process was first used to evaluate prevention programs, and has now been extended to treatment programs. The criteria are quite rigorous and include 18 methodological considerations (scientific rigor) and three appropriateness criteria.

The Methodological Criteria

Each criterion (beginning on page 44) is rated on a six-point scale as outlined below:

0 = non-applicable

1 = unacceptable

2 = poor

3 = fair

4 = very good

5 = excellent

Table 3.3   Practices Approved in Oregon as EBPs as of July 2006

- Substance Abuse
  - o 12-step facilitation (PDF) http://egov.oregon.gov/DHS/mentalhealth/ebp/ap/12step.pdf
  - o ASAM (PDF) http://egov.oregon.gov/DHS/mentalhealth/ebp/ap/asam.pdf
  - o Behavioral Couples (Marital) Therapy
  - o Behavioral Therapy for Adolescents
  - o Behavioral Therapy/Nicotine Replacement Therapy
  - o Brief Strategic Family Therapy http://egov.oregon.gov/DHS/mentalhealth/ebp/ap/practices.shtml.#dp
  - o Buprenorphine
  - o Cannabis Youth Treatment
  - o Cognitive Behavioral Therapy (CBT)—Depression in Adolescents (PDF) http://egov.oregon.gov/DHS/mentalhealth/ebp/ap/cbt-dep-adol.pdf
  - o CBT—Project Match (PDF) http://egov.oregon.gov/DHS/mentalhealth/ebp/ap/cbt.sa.pdf
  - o CBT—Trauma Focused (PDF) http://egov.oregon.gov/DHS/mentalhealth/ebp/ap/tfcbt.pdf
  - o Community Reinforcement Approach (CRA) with Vouchers
  - o Cognitive Behavioral Therapy for Child Sexual Abuse (CBT-CSA) (PDF) http://modelprograms.samhsa.gov/pdfs/FactSheet/CBT_CSA.pdf
  - o Co-Occurring Disorders: Integrated Dual Diagnosis Disorders (PDF) http:// egov.oregon.gov/DHS/mentalhealth/ebp/ap/iddt-application.pdf
  - o DBT Substance Abuse (PDF) http://egov.oregon.gov/DHS/mentalhealth/ebp/ap/dbt-sub-abuse.pdf
  - o Drug Court, Treatment Court, MH Courts, Family Courts
  - o Functional Family Therapy (PDF) http://egov.oregon.gov/DHS/mentalhealth/ebp/ap/fft.pdf
  - o Individual Drug Counseling
  - o Matrix Model (PDF) http://egov.oregon.gov/DHS/mentalhealth/ebp/ap/matrix.pdf
  - o Medication Management
  - o Moral Reconation Therapy
  - o Motivational Enhancement Therapy (MET) (PDF) http://egov.oregon.gov/DHS/mentalhealth/ebp/ap/met.pdf
  - o Motivational Interviewing (PDF) http://egov.oregon.gov/DHS/mentalhealth/ebp/ap/mot-int.pdf
  - o Multidimensional Family Therapy (PDF) http://egov.oregon.gov/DHS/mentalhealth/ebp/ap/Details/multi.pdf
  - o Multidimensional Treatment Foster Care (PDF) http://egov.oregon.gov/DHS/mentalhealth/ebp/ap/mtfc.pdf
  - o Multisystemic Family Therapy (PDF) http://egov.oregon.gov/DHS/mentalhealth/ebp/ap/multisys-fam-therapy.pdf
  - o Outpatient Treatment with Synthetic Opioid Replacement Therapy (Methadone) (PDF) http://egov.oregon.gov/DHS/mentalhealth/ebp/ap/methadone.pdf
  - o Relapse Prevention

(Continued)

Table 3.3 (Continued)

---

  o Seeking Safety (PDF) http://egov.oregon.gov/DHS/mentalhealth/ebp/ap/
    seek-safety.pdf
  o Wraparound (PDF) http://egov.oregon.gov/DHS/mentalhealth/ebp/ap/
    wraparound.pdf

- Co-Occurring Disorders
  o Co-Occurring Disorders: Integrated Dual Diagnosis Disorders (PDF)
    http://egov.oregon.gov/DHS/mentalhealth/ebp/iddt-application.pdf
  o DBT Substance Abuse (PDF) http://egov.oregon.gov/DHS/mentalhealth/ebp/
    ap/dbt-sub-abuse.pdf
  o Illness Management and Recovery (PDF) http://egov.oregon.gov/DHS/
    mentalhealth/ebp/ap/imr.pdf
  o Multidimensional Family Therapy (PDF) http://modelprograms.samhsa.gov/
    pdfs/Details/multi.pdf
  o Multidimensional Treatment Foster Care (PDF) http://egov.oregon.gov/DHS/
    mentalhealth/ebp/ap/mtfc.pdf
  o Seeking Safety (PDF) http://egov.oregon.gov/DHS/mentalhealth/ebp/ap/
    seek-safety.pdf

NOTE: The PDF after some practices indicates that they provide additional information on these practices, available on their Web sites: http://egov.oregon.gov/DHS/mentalhealth/ebp/main.shtml

Theory/Conceptual Underpinnings/Hypothesis: The degree to which the practice or program findings are consistent with a well-articulated theory with clearly stated hypotheses or a logical conceptual framework, and the extent to which the intervention activities and outcomes are linked to the theory or framework.

Intervention Fidelity: Evidence that fidelity implementation has been addressed.

Process Evaluation: The extent to which process evaluation methods were used to assess the implementation of the intervention, including contextual variables that explain findings, participation levels, success of outreach activities, and so on.

Research Design: The extent to which the research design was suitable for testing outcome effects. This criterion focuses on the acceptability of the control or comparison group.

Method of Group Assignment: This criterion assesses whether random assignment or other matching procedures were used.

Sample Size: Determines if the sample size was calculated using power analyses, and whether the sample size was adequate to answer the research questions.

Attrition: Sample dropout rates need to be noted. Attrition rates of less than 20 percent are considered ideal.

Analyses of Attrition Effects: This criterion assesses the appropriateness of the methods used to analyze attrition and account for attrition in the statistical analyses.

Methods of Correcting Biases: Bias can arise from non-equivalence of groups, attrition, or missing data. This criterion assesses the degree to which these issues are addressed or corrected.

Outcome Measures: Substantive Relevance: This criterion measures whether the study addressed the context of the target population, the theory or conceptual framework, and the intervention goals.

Outcome Measures: Psychometric Properties: The reliability and validity of the outcome measures are assessed.

Missing Data: The amount of missing data in the final data set.

Treatment of Missing Data: The degree to which missing data are analyzed adequately.

Outcome Data Collection: The quality of the procedures used to collect outcome data, including demand characteristics and whether the measures are standardized. This includes whether the outcome measures are collected in an anonymous or confidential manner, and the racial or ethnic and gender match between data collectors and clients.

Analysis Considerations: The technical adequacy of the statistical analyses.

Other Plausible Threats to Validity: The degree to which the research design and implementation address and eliminate alternative hypotheses or explanations for study findings, and the degree to which the study design allows for making statements about causality.

Integrity: The overall confidence in the findings based on the research methodology.

Utility: The overall usefulness of the findings to inform theory and practice, especially in regard to the strength of the findings and the evaluation.

The three appropriateness criteria include:

1. Replications: the number of replications and adaptations of the model (by age, gender, other adaptations) resulting in similar positive outcomes.

2. Dissemination Capability: whether there are training programs, manuals, technical assistance, standardized curriculum, evaluation materials, fidelity instruments, videos, and so on available to new users.

3. Cultural, Gender, and Age Appropriateness: the degree to which the program can be used across many populations.

Finally, the programs or practices are rated on three program descriptors.

1. Research design is included in the program description (whether they had pre-post tests, control groups, and so on).

2. A comparison/control group is included at all key data collection points.

3. The number of subjects at pretest, posttest, and final follow-up are reported for each group.

After all the ratings are completed, programs are placed in one of three categories, or not listed in the registry if there is insufficient support for use of the program or practice:

1. Model Programs and Practices have the highest level of scientific support, plus the capacity to be implemented easily into the field. There are 50 programs and practices already identified as model programs, mostly in the prevention field.

2. Effective Programs and Practices are scientifically sound, but may not be in a form that makes them easily implementable.

3. Promising Programs and Practices have some scientific support, but not sufficient to totally endorse them.

The Center for Substance Abuse Prevention (CSAP) has been using this system for a few years, and the Center for Substance Abuse Treatment (CSAT) has just begun using the system in the past year. Unfortunately, there are very few treatment practices listed in the registry, and the database, although searchable, is not very user-friendly. In late June 2006, SAMHSA officials outlined their priorities for review of practices and programs (*Federal Register*, 2006). All potential submissions must meet three minimum requirements:

1. The intervention must demonstrate one or more positive outcomes in mental health and/or substance abuse behaviors.

2. The intervention must be published in a peer-reviewed journal or in a comprehensive evaluation report.

3. Documentation must be available to the public in the form of manuals, implementation guides, training needs, materials, and so on.

SAMHSA estimated that it may take 3 to 5 years before the Web site is useful to the treatment field.

Conclusions

While SAMHSA is in the process of identifying effective programs and practices, there is, as of yet, no federal mandate to use evidence-based practices. Oregon is the only state with such a mandate. However, many states, regions, and individual agencies struggle to define best practices. At present, the NREPP criteria appear to be the most scientifically stringent set of measures, although they do allow for identification of promising practices with less scientific evidence available. NREPP puts the burden on the federal agency to evaluate practices and programs. Oregon's criteria put the onus on the individual provider agency to demonstrate that its officials are using evidence-based practices, although they are offering a significant amount of technical assistance. In Iowa, the criteria have been applied only in a pilot test and are not widely used in the state as of yet. They need to undergo testing for a weighting system before they are of practical use in the field. Until the science base is further developed, and researchers and providers work together to produce products that can be implemented in the field, mandates appear to be premature. The addendum to this chapter provides some guidance in developing criteria for a specific agency or region.

Addendum: Suggestions for Developing Criteria

The first question to ask is *Who needs to be involved in the process?* The number and type of people at the table to discuss the criteria will be keys to success in identifying good criteria and developing a process for implementing evidence-based practices. For example, Iowa established a committee consisting of substance abuse providers, policymakers, and researchers to develop the draft criteria, and then the criteria were reviewed by the statewide substance abuse program directors association and state-level policymakers. Commitment to evidence-based practice will require the establishment of an ongoing committee or task force that reviews new procedures. This group needs to include a few people with research expertise who have access to research reports and who will be able to evaluate the rigor of the research studies; a few people who thoroughly understand the practice arena and can advise the group on the practical issues of implementing the practice; and a few policymakers who are familiar with funding streams and payment systems.

To be effective, this committee will need to have some authority—will they advise some other decision-making body or have authority to select and enforce use of practices? There are different challenges if the decisions are top-down (some higher authority sets the criteria and selects the practices), bottom-up (line staff or agencies set the criteria and identify practices), or interdisciplinary (people from different disciplines and different levels in the hierarchy cooperate on the process).

Once the committee has been formed, here are a few points to consider:

- Who are the clients?
- What is currently being done? Are there any needs assessment or outcome data on the practices that are being used? What are the shortcomings of the current treatment approach, or what are the gaps in services?
- How much evidence is needed? If the goal is to identify one or two of the most highly researched practices, rigorous evidence is required. However, if the goal is to identify a broad range of practices with some research evidence to support them, the committee may be satisfied with looser criteria. The more evidence that is required, the more restricted the list of acceptable practices will be.
- Does the practice need to be manualized? Again, if this is the criterion, the number of acceptable practices will be small. On the other hand, if the practice is not manualized, someone at the agency level will have to do a lot of work to make it applicable to his or her setting. (This may be a good thing because the practice can be adapted to specific needs—but remember that with too much adaptation, it is no longer an evidence-based practice.)
- Does a practice have to meet all the criteria to be accepted? Will there be some kind of weighting system or score, or a set of required criteria and some that are optional? For the greatest flexibility, clinical practice guidelines may be more helpful than evidence-based practices.
- How much weight will be given to practical considerations relative to scientific merit? Is one more important than the other? In reality, the cost, availability, and acceptability to staff and clients may be of equal concern to scientific merit.

- Plan to examine outcome measures or indicators as part of the process of evaluating and adopting new practices. Different practices may require different forms of screening, assessment, and outcome evaluation. Build this discussion into the committee or task force from the beginning.
- Consider fidelity from the beginning. A practice may be practical and supported by research, but if it is difficult or too costly to measure its fidelity, it will have less value.
- Are trainers readily available in the area, or will the group have to expend considerable money in bringing in trainers or sending staff away for training?
- Research literature searches are time-consuming and potentially costly. The committee may need a research assistant, or a designated person to carry out searches.
- The research reports that describe the more rigorous research, such as randomized clinical trials or meta-analysis, are written with dense scientific jargon and multitudes of statistical terms. A researcher skilled in research design and statistics and skilled in translating that information into plain English is an essential member of the committee.

4

Adoption and Implementation of Evidence-Based Practices

Despite decades of evidence supporting the efficacy of behaviorally oriented couples counseling, only 4% of substance abuse treatment programs reported using it (Fals-Stewart & Birchler, 2001). . . . This gap is perpetuated to the extent that internship and degree programs preparing the next generation of substance abuse professionals continue to neglect evidence-based treatment in training. Graduate programs and internships in psychology . . . may not require students to develop competence in even one empirically validated treatment (Crits-Christoph, Frank, Chambless, Brody, & Karp, 1995), if indeed they address addictions at all during clinical training. (Miller & Brown, 1997; Miller et al., 2006, p. 26)

The quotation above highlights the tremendous challenges facing the evidence-based practice movement. Once a practice has been sufficiently studied, evaluated with acceptable scientific rigor, and found to be significantly better than treatment as usual, how does it get into the field? Significant changes in the way the field does business—from counselor training to agency mission statements and hiring practices to clinical supervision models and fidelity measurement systems—are needed to accommodate the new evidence-based practice model. "Build it and they will come" may have worked in the movies, but in real life, many factors influence adoption and implementation of a new practice. There is much more research on the efficacy of certain treatment approaches than on how to implement those approaches in a clinical practice. Backer (1993) suggested that for a new

51

approach to be implemented, first it must have evidence to support its use. Then it must be put into a form for dissemination, agencies must be made aware of the approach, they must have resources to implement it, and interventions must be developed that encourage and enable agencies to change their current procedures to incorporate the new innovation. Current approaches of disseminating research information are geared toward researchers, such as conference presentations and journal articles. However, merely translating research into manuals or practice guidelines does not ensure implementation. Organizational factors that influence adoption and implementation must be considered. Risk-taking leaders of agencies may be quick to decide to adopt new practices, but line staff, with lower pay, high burnout, and often less education, are the ones expected to implement the practice. Both agency directors and line staff must be taken into account in an implementation plan. Change leaders or opinion leaders, those staff members who are enthusiastic about a new approach and respected by their peers, are a necessary ingredient in the adoption phase.

Assessment of Readiness to Change

Training is expensive and time-consuming, so it is important to determine if it is feasible to introduce a new treatment approach before launching a training program. Lehman, Greener, and Simpson (2002) described an instrument for assessing program director and line staff readiness to change. This instrument is available for free from the Texas Christian University Web site (www.ibr.tcu.edu). It has two forms—one for leaders of the organization and one for treatment staff. The instrument has 115 items in four scales:

1. Motivational readiness
   a. Perceived program needs for improvement
   b. Training needs
   c. Pressure for change

2. Institutional resources
   a. Office
   b. Staffing
   c. Training resources
   d. Computer access
   e. Electronic communications

3. Staff attributes
   a. Value placed on professional growth
   b. Efficacy (confidence in counseling skills)

     c. Willingness and ability to influence coworkers
     d. Adaptability

  4. Organizational climate
     a. Clarity of mission and goals
     b. Staff cohesiveness
     c. Staff autonomy
     d. Openness of communication
     e. Level of stress
     f. Openness to change

The problem with such a scale is that someone must administer it and enter and analyze the data. Smaller agencies may prefer to work through open discussions with staff about potential changes and seek consensus for decisions to adopt a new procedure.

Instituting Organizational Change

Dwayne Simpson (2002) proposed a four-factor model of program change, outlined in simplified form in Table 4.1. Once a program has been assessed and considered "ready to change," the process would begin with exposure, or

Table 4.1   Simpson's Model of Program Change

Factor	Description	Influences
Exposure	Training (lectures, self-study, workshops, consultation)	Motivation of leaders and staff, institutional resources (staffing, facilities, training, equipment), and convenience of training
Adoption	Intention to try the new approach	Motivational readiness, group versus individual decision to adopt, reception and utility of the approach (adequacy of training, ease of use, fit into value system of the individual or agency)
Implementation	Trial use	Support of institution, addition of resources, climate for change, rewards for change
Practice	Sustaining the new practice over time	Staff attributes (self-efficacy, professional growth, adaptability)

training. Training can be the traditional one-shot workshop approach—if the new procedure is a simple technique—or a highly concrete manual, or can be ongoing and multimodal if the new innovation entails a major change in philosophy or involves complex techniques or procedures. However, as the model indicates, exposure alone does not ensure adoption; indeed, it is only the first step. Agencies and individuals must intend to try the approach, actually implement it, and then make its use regular and embedded in daily practice.

Exposure includes three critical factors. The first is motivation, or the perceived need for change and/or pressure to change, from individual staff members as well as program leaders. The second factor is resources. There must be sufficient staffing, training, facilities, and equipment to carry out the intervention. Finally, convenience of training is important—are the time, location, and the ease of the training format conducive to engagement?

If there was no motivation during the exposure phase, then the process stops. However, if we assume that motivation was present, decisions about adoption are made next. This can be at the line staff level if the counselor finds the practice worthwhile and incorporates it into his or her daily practice, or adoption can occur at the larger program or agency level, where staff members collectively decide to adopt. Adoption decisions are influenced by reception and perceived utility of the practice, including such factors as the adequacy of the training, the perceived ease of adoption, and how well the practice fits into the treatment philosophy and mission of the agency and the individual staff.

Implementation begins when a decision has been made to adopt the practice. If adequate resources are identified and the climate is conducive to change, then the agency or program is ready. The climate for change consists of many factors, such as the clarity of the mission and goals of the program, staff cohesion, degree of clinical autonomy, styles of communication, general level of stress, and whether there is an openness to change in the program. Institutional support in the form of monitoring and supervision, feedback, and provision of rewards for change are needed to maintain the enthusiasm for implementation.

Finally, in the practice phase, the incorporation of the new approach into daily practice depends on staff attributes such as commitment to professional growth, efficacy, and adaptability as well as on continued institutional support for the practice, including feedback and reward.

Challenges to Implementation

The practical consideration items in the Iowa criteria and the appropriateness criteria of the National Registry of Evidence-Based Programs and

Practices (NREPP) were developed with adoption and implementation of new practices in mind. If a practice is not acceptable to staff, clients, or the community at large, if it is not in a form that is easily adapted to the field, or if it is too expensive, it will not be adopted no matter how effective it might be. Box 4.1 gives the example of naltrexone—a drug highly supported by research, but rarely used in practice. However, even practices that meet all the practicality criteria will present challenges to implementation. The potential barriers to implementation of a new practice are reviewed below. They include training issues; individual variation in clients, staff, and agencies; buy-in; commitment; negative attitudes about research; lack of research-practice partnerships; lack of resources; and organizational factors.

Box 4.1   An Example of Lack of Implementation: Naltrexone

Naltrexone was approved in 1994, and is quite effective, safe, and easy to administer. There is considerable research, including several clinical trials and at least two meta-analyses, that shows its effectiveness on reducing heavy drinking and reducing severity of relapse. In addition to the voluminous research literature, there is a CSAT TIP (O'Malley, 1998) that gives clinical guidance for using it in treatment. So is it widely used in practice? Roman and Johnson (2002) reported that only 5 percent of substance abuse counselors routinely recommended it to eligible clients and more than half (54 percent) never recommended it. That seems understandable, given that naltrexone is a medication that is prescribed by a doctor and therefore substance abuse counselors would not be as likely to give buy-in, as well as the fact that it is contrary to the core beliefs of some counselors that no medications should be used to treat addictions. How about physicians? A study of members of the American Society of Addiction Medicine, the group of physicians most likely to know about and use naltrexone, reported that they prescribed it for only about 13 percent of their clients (Mark et al., 2003). The main impetus for prescribing naltrexone seemed to be if the organization promoted it and if insurance or Medicaid paid for it.

Training Issues

The Veteran's Affairs system recently reviewed nine experimental studies about adoption of new practices into the clinical work of physicians. They concluded that distributing print materials and conducting the typical continuing education lecture program had virtually no impact on clinical practice (Backer, 2003). Clearly we need new models for training. Research has suggested that training must be ongoing, not a one-shot, hit-and-run activity. There are a number of reasons why training must take place over time:

1. Complex learning does not occur in one session—training of new skills must occur over time so that learners can practice the skill in a real-life setting and work through any problems with the trainers and experts. Supervision (or individual coaching) and feedback are two critical components of learning a new practice (Miller et al., 2004; Morgenstern et al., 2001).

2. Learning must be reinforced frequently. Even the fastest learners tend to drift back to old practices over time if the new skills are not reinforced. This process of drift from protocol needs more study (Miller et al., 2006) and may be addressed by having onsite experts or by regular contact with outside consultants by phone, the Web, or other technology.

3. Some new practices require a shift in provider attitudes in addition to learning new skills. Attitude change takes time. Workshops may jump-start attitude change (Hayes et al., 2004; McCarty et al., 2004), but follow-up contact is necessary to translate attitude change to behavior change (Sholomskas et al., 2005; Sorensen et al., 1988). For some staff members, attitude change will not occur until they observe the impact in their own agencies or on their own clients.

4. There is considerable staff turnover in the field, with a continual need to train new staff. Staff turnover rates of about one third of the staff per year are common in substance abuse agencies, meaning that ongoing training of new staff is critical.

Sorensen and colleagues (1988) found that even when they provided onsite personal consultation about a new approach, 72 percent of agencies failed to fully implement the program. If they merely provided manuals, 96 percent failed to implement the program fully. So what is needed? It seems that effective trainers, good materials, training conducted over a period of time, and varied formats for training are components of technology transfer.

Who should conduct the training? Often the researchers who develop new interventions are not skilled in training others to use it, and lack incentives from their departments to engage in extensive training activities. Very often the development of the manuals and training programs comes from their professional staff, individuals with clinical experience who have worked with the research team.

There is no consensus on the best way to deliver training. In fact, in recent years, experts have realized that our old training models are inadequate to the task of getting research into practice. Recent models focus on technology transfer, a broader process of moving the field to accept change, incorporate science into practice, and maintain change over time. Technology transfer involves not only training of new skills, but builds in motivation or incentives to change and considers the organizational issues that inhibit or facilitate change.

Training is a major tool of technology transfer. Most staff still prefer face-to-face, workshop-style training. However, cost and time considerations have led to an increase in distance learning technologies. Some suggestions for improving the training of new practices include:

Develop a Plan: An extensive training and technology transfer plan early on will guide the process in a more systematic manner. As soon as evidence-based practices are identified, consider:

- How best to institute training (face-to-face, online, videoconference).
- How many people need to be trained.
- Whether effective trainers or materials are available in the area at low cost.
- How long the initial training must be.
- What format the training will take (self-study, videotapes, workshops, and so on).
- When refresher, reinforcer, or advanced training courses will be offered.
- How model fidelity will be addressed.

Use Varied Learning Formats: Use a variety of learning formats to increase the chance of reaching as many counselors as possible:

- Face-to-face
- Self-study
- Videoconferencing
- CD-ROM or DVD
- Videotapes or audiotapes
- Conference calls

Train Teams: Train teams rather than individuals—they can support each other when they return to their agencies or programs.

"Train the Trainer": Select opinion leaders (staff members who are highly influential among their peers) or clinical supervisors and train them in the new practice. They in turn train other members of their staff and supervise the implementation of the new practice. These trainers need backup and support in their agencies. Training and supervision need to be built into job descriptions rather than being added-on duties.

Use Manual Driven Training: Use existing manuals or develop treatment manuals, and train staff from the manuals. While knowing the theoretical background of an approach is important, most of the training should focus on direct concrete skills. The more direct the learning, the greater the fidelity will be.

Train Key Administrative Staff: Make sure that program directors and clinical supervisors have been trained. If only line staff are sent to training, they may not receive adequate support, understanding, or supervision to maintain the new practice.

Build Practice Time Into the Training Plan: For example, there may be a week-long initial training, followed by three monthly consultations or case conferences to reinforce the learning and discuss any difficulties that arose when staff implemented the practice. Alternatively, the training can be staged with initial training followed by time to practice the skills in real life, then by more advanced training or reinforcement of the skills in a few months.

Have Pretraining Requirements: For example, require participants to view videos; read a book, articles, or manuals; take a survey; do a self-assessment; and so on. Theoretically, participants will then come to the training with a baseline of knowledge.

Offer Incentives for Learning the New Skill: Provide certificates, continuing education credit, money, or promotions and/or make it prestigious.

Client Variation

There are a variety of individual factors that may affect implementation, including client, staff, and agency diversity. First, there are client variations. For example, some clients do not have the cognitive abilities to benefit from some cognitive-behavioral or insight-oriented practices. Some clients are unable to read, and many have learning and attention disorders that may impact their ability to engage with certain types of therapeutic practices. Other clients may object to the religious or spiritual basis of some practices. Physically disabled clients may not be able to participate in some kinds of group activities. Drug use patterns fluctuate with the availability of substances, and treatment services today may not meet the client needs of tomorrow. For example, do methamphetamine users benefit from the same practices that are effective for opioid users? Clients from minority groups may not relate as well to materials developed for majority clients, and vice versa. Client diversity must be considered when selecting practices, and/or contingency plans for how to deal with clients who are unable to engage in the practice must be developed. If staff perceive too many barriers to using this practice with their clients, they are not likely to be motivated to learn the new skills.

Provider/Staff Variation

There are also variations in provider attitudes and skills. Some staff members may refuse or be unable to learn the skills of one type of practice. Some new innovations fit well with a staff member's existing treatment approach, whereas others present major challenges to the counselor's usual practice. Staff members vary on the value they place on professional growth, their degree of investment in one way of providing treatment, their adaptability, and a host of other factors that may influence whether they adopt the practice or not. For example, some line staff have little formal education, but learned counseling techniques through their own recovery—nearly half of substance abuse counselors in the late 1980s (Mulligan, McCarty, Potter, & Krakow, 1985) and about 40 percent currently (Eliason et al., 2005; McGovern, Fox, Xie, & Drake, 2004). If they recovered in a highly confrontational type of program they may resist practices such as motivational interviewing. Other practices, such as dialectical therapy for clients with borderline personality disorder, may require staff with a high degree of education and a commitment to learning complex skills. Many agencies cannot afford to hire staff with higher education, or when they do, they quickly take on supervisory or administrative roles and have limited clinical duties.

Ball et al. (2002) were interested in whether counselor theoretical orientation might be a factor in whether they could be trained to some new practice. They studied counselors who volunteered to participate in motivational interviewing (MI) and motivational enhancement therapy (MET) studies in the Clinical Trials Network. They chose counselors who had not had recent or extensive training in MI/MET and gathered information on their demographic backgrounds and treatment philosophies. They reported that most of these counselors endorsed a cognitive behavioral (78 percent) or 12-step model (55 percent), whereas fewer endorsed MI (34 percent) or Rogerian counseling (44 percent). However, their specific beliefs about treatment were most consistent with a directive style and an abstinence outcome, suggesting that they might be resistant to MI/MET training. It will be interesting to note the final results of this study—who was successfully trained in MI/MET?

Dwayne Simpson and colleagues (Institute of Behavioral Research, 2001/ 2002) also studied counselor characteristics and adoption of new practices. They offered workshops on highly specific and concrete practices, including distribution of manuals, then followed up on how many participants actually used the materials. More than 67 percent of counselors used an assessment manual; 52 percent used a gender-specific communication/sexual health manual; 46 percent used the contingency management materials; and 25 percent reported implementing a cognitive strategies manual. The counselors who had not used the materials and reported no intention of using them gave these reasons: lack of time, lack of resources to implement the materials, they already used similar materials, and poor fit with their personal counseling style.

Program/Agency Variation

There are also variations in agencies—they vary in physical environment, age and stability, geographic region, layout, location ("bad" neighborhood, inaccessible), philosophy, access to health care providers or mental health resources, funding sources, longevity and characteristics of the executive director, composition and engagement by board members, and a host of other variables. Knudsen and Roman (2004) suggested that organizations vary in "absorptive capacity," or the ability to access and effectively use information. They found that agencies that were good at environmental scanning (using informational resources such as professional development seminars and publications) and those that routinely collected satisfaction data were more likely to adopt new innovations than agencies that were low on these dimensions. Building capacity in these areas will increase the speed of adoption of evidence-based practices (EBPs).

Take these program/agency factors into account when establishing criteria and identifying new practices:

- Specify who the clients are before selecting practices and keep their needs in mind while reviewing potential practices.
- Develop policies for implementation—is the new practice mandatory or voluntary? If mandatory, there must be clearly articulated policies for completion of training, use of the practice, and fidelity measurement. If use of the practice is not mandatory, will it be confusing to clients if some staff use the practice and others do not? Some treatment philosophies are compatible with each other, whereas others are not. For example, if some counselors use practices to break down denial, and others "roll with resistance," will clients react negatively?
- Will all of the programs use the new practice, or only some of the programs or components of programs?
- Assess the workplace or agency climate: Does the practice match the treatment philosophy or mission of the agency? Can it logistically work in this environment? Are there a sufficient number of staff to conduct the treatment program?

Buy-In

In order to effectively implement a new practice, there must be sufficient support at all levels: from the funding source, the board of directors, the agency director, clinical supervisors, line staff, receptionists and other staff, clients, and the community.

- Involve key stakeholders in the process from the beginning.
- Introduce the idea gradually or in definable phases—keep all staff informed of the work of the committee or workgroup.
- Elicit input from staff at major decision points.
- Use opinion leaders—identify key staff or clients who are influential among their peers and train them in the new practice first (Valente, 2002). Peters et al. (2005) found that counselors who attended opinion leader–facilitated training were more likely to implement and use a new practice than counselors who got typical training. Opinion leaders can become ambassadors for the new approach. Some agency directors may think that they know who the opinion leaders are in their agencies, but could be wrong. Staff may have different attitudes about their coworkers. If opinion leaders are used, do some assessment of staff to find out who those leaders really are.

Commitment

Buy-in is only the first step to implementation. Once a new practice is identified, the funding source, agency directors, and clinical supervisors must make a commitment to the practice. This commitment involves devoting a certain amount of time to the new practice so that it can be adequately implemented and evaluated. It also includes a commitment to training, supervision, and monitoring of the practice. Far too often, agencies have enthusiastically adopted a new practice, but abandoned it within months when obstacles were encountered. The temptation to switch approaches is strong—there are many charismatic presenters at conferences or new treatment manuals in the mail. If there is no long-term commitment, do not even attempt the process of implementing evidence-based practices.

Negative Attitudes/Lack of Knowledge About Research

Many providers and policymakers have little or no training in research methods, and some have negative attitudes about research. There is a prevailing myth that substance abuse treatment is largely a self-help movement that does not need professional intervention or scientifically based treatments. Even providers who have positive attitudes about research often do not have the skills to interpret research findings in their traditional forms—in research journals, monographs, or evaluation reports. Some suggestions for changing attitudes and knowledge about research include:

Researcher-in-Residence Programs: Have a researcher meet with staff in the treatment agencies to discuss research findings or evidence-based practices. This may increase the communication between researchers and providers as well as foster more positive attitudes. Choose a researcher who has the ability to communicate with nonresearchers and who is willing to meet providers on their own turf.

Designated Research Staff Member: Assign one (willing) staff member to write research briefs for a newsletter or bulletin board. These news briefs or summaries of research are already available from a variety of sources, such as the Join Together Web site (www.jointogether.org/), the Addiction Technology Transfer Centers Web sites and newsletters (www.nattc.org/index.html), and the Center for Substance Abuse Research (CESAR: www.cesar.umd.edu/).

Continuing Education/Inservice: Seek continuing education programs, inservice programs, or guest speakers who introduce research concepts or share their experiences with new practices.

Conferences: Send staff members to research-oriented conferences with the requirement that they report back on what they learned in staff meetings and share good materials with others.

Discussion/Reading Groups: Start a journal club and discuss research studies or issues with other staff. This potentially instills a research-positive climate for the agency.

Pilot Studies: Involve staff in small-scale research projects in the agency or region by including them on committees or teams to conduct needs assessments, measure outcomes, or address other treatment issues. The practice improvement method of testing "rapid cycle" changes is also a good way to introduce a simple form of research process (see the NIATx Web site http://chess.chsra.wisc.edu/NIATx/Home/ for suggestions).

Lack of Practice-Research Partnerships/Collaborations

Service providers must be involved in setting research agendas and be active participants in applied research. Researchers need to find nontraditional ways to disseminate their research findings so that they are relevant and applicable to the field. Policymakers need to base policy decisions on research, not on public opinion. The only way that these problems can be solved is through collaborations. The National Treatment Plan (CSAT, 2000) outlined the relationships among the three major components of substance abuse treatment research:

1. Knowledge Development consists of applied and basic research, such as that generated by the National Institute on Drug Abuse (NIDA), the National Institute on Alcoholism and Alcohol Abuse (NIAAA), the Centers for Disease Control and Prevention (CDC), and investigator-driven research studies.

2. Knowledge Transfer is the dissemination of knowledge in the form of training, changing attitudes, behaviors, and skills, such as the activities of Addiction Technology Transfer Centers and the Center for Substance Abuse Treatment (CSAT) Treatment Improvement Protocols (TIPs).

3. Knowledge Application consists of learning how to implement new practices into the field. This is the newest of the three components of research, so we have less guidance in this area.

For any of these three components to work, collaborations across the funding agencies, service delivery systems, and state, county, and regional substance abuse treatment arenas must be developed. All three components inform each other. The activities of practice-research collaboratives can include:

- Publication of research findings in diverse formats accessible to providers, such as newsletters, manuals, e-mail or fax briefs, assessment tools, and so on. Researchers do not benefit from developing such publications, so this may require working with a staff member who is able to translate the research into practical products, or using national programs such as Join Together or the Addiction Technology Transfer Centers to find these materials.
- Technical assistance in implementing new practices and evaluating outcomes.
- Developing studies that focus on the adoption of new practices.

Successful collaborations are like an intimate relationship. First there is a period of trust-building, feeling out each other's values, goals, and agenda, and developing a common language. Then roles can be negotiated, and commitment to a longer-term relationship can be made. Box 4.2 gives examples of questions that providers can ask of researchers to determine if they might be a good match.

Box 4.2   Interviewing Researchers

The Institute of Medicine report (Lamb, Greenlick, & McCarty, 1998) listed 10 questions that providers could ask researchers to identify those willing to collaborate with them (offered from provider Chilo Madrid of El Paso, Texas). The questions include the following:

1. What funds are available for clinical services? Does the entire budget go to research?
2. Are the researchers sensitive to cultural issues in the agency?
3. Will the study address questions that are applicable to my agency?
4. Are the research questions practical? Will the purpose of the study be explained, or is deception (such as placebo treatments) involved?
5. How will my agency benefit from participating? What kind of technical assistance, training, or other benefits may accrue?
6. Are there potential risks to clients, beyond the ones involved in any treatment?
7. What might be the long-term benefits for the program or agency?
8. Does the researcher express genuine concern for the program and its clients?
9. How much choice does the program have in the selection of the researcher or the research team members with whom to work?
10. If there is a separate evaluation, does the program have a say in choosing the evaluator?

Broner, Franczak, Dye, and McAllister (2001) proposed an empowerment, consensus model for research-practice collaboratives that is aimed at "co-creation" of knowledge. This model requires a major paradigm shift from the old ways. Traditional knowledge production models assume that knowledge flows from the experts in empirical science down to the practitioners, and learning is considered a simple matter of instruction. This old model fails to recognize the critical role of the end-user of the knowledge. When end-users work in consensus-building activities with researchers, with an expectation that all members of the collaboration are experts in different aspects of the issue, co-created knowledge results. This type of knowledge will theoretically be easier to implement in real-world settings. Broner et al. (2001) suggested four mechanisms for establishing these research-practice partnerships:

1. Use "bridgers," or leaders who are capable of bringing together the diverse stakeholders who are needed for a production collaboration. A bridger is

respected by all the stakeholders and is skilled in communication and conflict resolution.

2. Establish community ownership of the end results by a broad and inclusive membership in the partnership. The "evidence" produced by this inclusive group belongs to the whole community.

3. Implement a consensus-building process with a specific method, workplan, and evaluation. Do not think the process will happen naturally.

4. Maintain the work by disseminating findings and reintegrating information. Look for multiple ways to continue the dialogue.

This model closely resembles the strategies of NIDA's Clinical Trials Network, where researchers and providers work together to identify the research agenda, design studies, develop protocols and training materials, and interpret findings.

Lack of Resources

Drug treatment programs are supported by a variety of different funding sources, including block grants, Medicaid, private insurance, state and local funding, and private donations. Each source may have different regulations about what services they will pay for. Perhaps the greatest obstacle to implementing evidence-based practices is the lack of resources, and the question of whether the various payment sources will support the new practice. Resources include money, staff, computers, space, and materials, among others. Substance abuse treatment agencies have always been underfunded and have always had to seek creative ways to provide services. Some of the ways to increase resources include the following.

Develop Partnerships: A variety of partners can be beneficial to the process of improving substance abuse treatment services. Three types of partnerships are described below:

- Partnerships with researchers who will write grants to provide services and do applied research that will benefit the agency and the field. This requires a good match between provider needs and researcher expertise. The partnership must be mutually beneficial. Most researchers are specialists in a particular area and are not willing or able to address a wide range of topics.
- Partnerships with businesses that may provide material goods, such as computers, training programs, photocopying, client incentives, transportation, and so on. For example, if an agency wants to try contingency management, the

incentives do not have to be money or be costly—small gift certificates to grocery stores or arcades may be donated.
- Partner with media agencies or individual reporters to publicize the good work the agency does.

Develop Community Volunteer Programs: These can be particularly helpful in identifying individuals from minority or underrepresented groups to consult about cultural competence, and can help improve community relationships and enhance buy-in to new practices, as well as provide volunteers or resources to fund a new program or practice. In addition, use fundraisers from the community—get at least one on your board of directors.

Designate a Research Liaison Staff Member: One (willing) staff member, preferably one who is an opinion leader, could serve as the grant writer and research coordinator. Send this person to workshops on grant writing.

Start With Free or Low-Cost Options: Consider starting with the evidence-based practices for which there are free materials, such as the manuals available online or by mail from CSAT, NIDA, or Texas Christian University.

Organizational Structure

Adoption and implementation often depend on factors directly related to the organizational structure, such as leadership (the agency director's training, education, treatment philosophy, vision, and creativity), caseload and staffing patterns, decision-making mechanisms, language (client versus patient, counselor versus therapist), and cultures and subcultures of the agency. Hospital-based programs differ from community-based programs in many ways, and may be more likely to readily adopt medically based approaches such as pharmacological treatments. Community-based programs may be more likely to consider group-based psychoeducational treatments because of staffing patterns, staff educational levels, and organizational philosophy.

The age of the organization may be an important factor. Older agencies are more likely to have a well-defined philosophy or mission statement and become more entrenched in their approach, and thus less likely to adopt new approaches than newer programs still under development (Rogers, 1995). Conversely, the older agency may be more stable and thus better equipped to try out new approaches because of a stable workforce. The length of time the director has been in place may also be important, as well as the educational degrees and level or type of training of the director. A director with a business background may provide different leadership than one with a mental health or substance abuse background.

The size of the agency may also be important, because larger agencies generally have more resources and greater flexibility to rearrange those resources. The percentage of staff with a master's degree or higher influences adoption, as staff members with higher education are more likely to have been exposed to research methods and research findings. The profit status of the agency may also be important. Private agencies may be less likely to consider new approaches that might temporarily disrupt patient flow. On the other hand, managed care contracts often demand that the most cost-effective treatments be provided (Roman, Johnson, & Blum, 2000). Finally, agencies with higher client relapse rates may be more open to change and to trying new approaches than agencies that perceive their relapse rate as acceptable (or do not keep data about outcomes at all).

Resources for data management affect the ability to track outcomes. Many agencies cannot afford to do follow-up on clients after they leave their programs. Sophisticated, Web-based tracking systems are available in business, but may be too expensive for community agencies. Some agencies collect only the data that are required by the county or state, whereas others are committed to monitoring a broad range of outcomes.

The Practice Itself

The complexity and other features of the new practice may also serve as a barrier to adoption. Rogers (1995) suggested five factors that predict whether a new practice might be implemented:

1. Relative advantage: the practice is perceived as being superior to existing practices.

2. Compatibility: the practice fits the individual and agency beliefs and values.

3. Complexity: The practice is fairly easy to understand and implement. Of the widely recognized evidence-based practices, some are fairly simple (giving a pill), whereas others require staff to master complex skills (dialectical behavioral therapy, motivational interviewing).

4. Trialability: the practice can be studied experimentally (researchers care about this; providers may not).

5. Observability: the practice can easily be seen by others. Obvious practices with visible outcomes are noticed by all staff.

An example is the Clinical Trials Network (CTN) efforts to test motivational interviewing. Carroll et al. (2002) described the steps and processes that went into designing a study of the effectiveness of MI in increasing treatment engagement and thus retaining clients in treatment. Aspects of the practice itself had to be taken into account. For example, the prior clinical trials had been on individual administration of one to five sessions of MI. In some treatment programs in the CTN, it was feasible to have several individual sessions with clients, whereas in other programs, clients had only one individual appointment, and went thereafter into treatment groups. Most of the earlier trials, and hence, the existing treatment manuals, focused on alcohol or tobacco; so manuals had to be rewritten to accommodate the wide diversity of client drug patterns. Most of the earlier trials had used highly educated, highly trained, and closely supervised therapists to deliver the intervention—very unlike the staff in most treatment programs. Could the typical substance abuse counselor learn and implement MI? What about potential volunteer bias if counselors were asked to nominate themselves for MI training?

Carroll et al. (2002) also noted that many treatment agencies had a treatment philosophy that was contrary to the nonjudgmental, empathic, collaborative approach of MI; and most earlier trials had excluded clients with co-occurring disorders and criminal justice involvement, making the samples atypical of the client base of most treatment agencies. Would MI work with these more difficult clients?

Other issues had to do with counselors' experiences. When presented with the basic descriptions of MI, many counselors reported that they already used the principles and techniques of MI, but review of their therapy audiotapes indicated otherwise. How would they deal with feedback that they were off the mark? Finally, most counselors had no experience using treatment manuals. In short, considerable training about the practice itself had to be done to accommodate all these differences from earlier trials in tightly controlled environments to the CTN, a situation closer to real life.

Stigma

The final barrier to adoption is related to stigma. Stigma pervades the substance abuse treatment field and can interfere with implementation of new practices in many ways. Community attitudes about treatment (the myth that treatment does not work), community attitudes about providers (misconceptions that they are all recovering addicts who cannot get work elsewhere), and attitudes about clients (they are willfully engaging in dangerous behavior) may lead to difficulty in placing programs in communities that need them (NIH, 1997). Methadone clinics and halfway houses are particularly hard to sell in residential areas. Stigma has also led to a lack of training in substance abuse in most health and human services educational programs, meaning that it is difficult to find physicians, nurses, psychologists, social workers, and educators with adequate education in substance abuse to staff new programs. Stigma affects the flow of federal, state, and local dollars in the proportions spent on treatment and prevention versus law enforcement and fighting the "war on drugs." Stigma has led to the incarceration of many substance abusers and the attitude that they require punishment rather than treatment. Substance abuse treatment providers, researchers, and local- and state-level policymakers need to become stronger political advocates for treatment.

Some potential ways to reduce stigma include:

- Volunteer to give talks in college and university classes in psychology, nursing, medical schools, social work programs, criminal justice programs, and so on. This may also serve to identify potential academic partners.
- Empower clients, and particularly those with greater periods of recovery, to speak up about policies that are discriminatory, and to become open role models in the community. Agencies might even offer classes or groups on advocacy issues for staff and mentors.
- Expand the base of the recovery community to include as many aspects of the larger community as possible. For example, elicit support from business leaders; faith communities; ethnic minority community leaders and organizations; women's groups; social service agencies; lesbian, gay, bisexual, and transgender organizations; and schools.
- Run for political office.

Conclusions

In conclusion, there is very little empirical research on the best ways to implement new practices in the field. Models of technology transfer or diffusion of innovation (such as those of Dwayne Simpson and Everett Rogers) are very helpful and need much more study. We do know that the old standby of training, the face-to-face, one-shot workshop, is a highly inefficient method of getting research into practice. Instead, we need a sustained effort at several levels addressing all the barriers to implementation in order to get new practices into the field and maintain their use over time.

This chapter has focused on individual and agency-level factors associated with adoption of evidence-based practices, but this may be too limiting. In the medical field, changes in financing (that is, paying for use of EBPs and not paying or paying less for unproven therapies) is the most effective way to effect rapid change in clinical practice (Sechrest et al., 1994). The experience in Oregon may give us some idea whether this is a viable option for the substance abuse treatment field.

5

Evaluation of Evidence-Based Practices

O nce the advantages of implementing evidence-based treatment practices are recognized, providers and policymakers often ask: *Why evaluate evidence-based approaches—after all, haven't they already been proven?* Put simply, it may be *even more important* to evaluate evidence-based practices. The effectiveness of an evidence-based treatment depends on faithful and complete implementation. There are many reasons why a program or practice may not be implemented precisely as written, but these deviations must be documented in order to either understand why the program was less effective than expected or report back to the field that certain deviations did not impact effectiveness or maybe even improved outcomes.

There are many lessons to be learned about how treatment programs work (or do not work) with specific populations or under unique circumstances—evaluating the program and reporting the results gives practitioners a chance to provide feedback and help refine the research base. This contributes to the practice-based evidence literature. Issues of client diversity can be addressed as well by observing whether the practice works better for some clients than others. If programs do not achieve intended outcomes, it is important to be able to tease out whether or not the program was fully implemented or if other factors account for the lack of positive outcomes.

Another reason to evaluate evidence-based practices is to ensure quality control and reduce program "drift," thereby retaining the full effect of evidence-based practices. However, it is sometimes necessary for programs to shift course slightly from established protocols due to cultural or linguistic population differences or unavoidable environmental circumstances (e.g., if a large health maintenance organization [HMO] reduces the number of treatment days it will pay for). In this case, the program needs to understand whether or not the changes they made in the evidence-based practice affected outcomes.

Evidence-based practices may have been proven effective in a particular place (e.g., a large treatment agency on the East Coast), for a particular mix of clients (e.g., men in a VA hospital opioid treatment program), and implemented by a particular group of counselors (who may have received extensive training by the research team, or were hand-picked as the "best" counselors at the agency). There are many examples in the medical literature of procedures that work very well in the laboratory, but do not produce the same results in a physician's office. The same is true of substance abuse treatment research. The field simply cannot know if the practice works unless evaluation data are collected. Accepting that something works on faith or other people's research is counter to the whole idea of evidence-based practice.

Study after study has shown that strong and positive client outcomes result when programs *accurately* implement evidence-based protocols (e.g., Jerrell & Ridgely, 1999; Mattson et al., 1998; McHugo, Drake, Teague, & Xie, 1999). This premise has been shown to be true not only in the field of substance abuse treatment but also in cardiovascular health (McGraw et al., 1996), criminal justice (Blakely, Mayer, & Gottschalk, 1987), and employment (McDonnell, Nofs, & Hardman, 1989). Understanding the integrity of program implementation also means that researchers and practitioners can have greater confidence in evaluation results. For example, evaluators studying the results of a smoking prevention program aimed at youth were able to report *with confidence* that the program had no effect on long-term smoking behaviors because they could show that the program had been rigorously implemented. In this example, the incorporation of fidelity measures into the evaluation gave the researchers a much better understanding of why the intervention did not work. In this case, it was not due to implementation failure, but due instead to flawed theory and design.

There are two main components of evaluations of evidence-based treatment programs: (1) *process evaluation* (or documentation of fidelity) and (2) *outcome evaluation* (did the program change behaviors?). These two very different kinds of evaluation are described in the following sections, along with a brief discussion of program evaluation.

Process Evaluation (Fidelity)

While process evaluation typically focuses on the characteristics of participants and the frequency and intensity—or dosage—of the intervention (often referred to as "reach and freq"), an assessment of fidelity adds value when evaluating evidence-based programs. Fidelity is "the degree to which a program's implementation matches the intended one" (Valente, 2002). Fidelity can be lost when treatment staff members do not apply the techniques of the evidence-based practice as they were trained. Programs often lose their fidelity to protocols over time or when they are implemented in unique settings. As programs grow and evolve, they may change in unexpected ways that can reduce effectiveness. This program "drift" is not always negative—some programs improve on outcomes because they are able to adapt successfully to local needs. Whether drift results in stronger or weaker outcomes, it is important to be able to report these findings back to the field so that other programs can gain from the lessons learned.

Because substance abuse treatment programs are notoriously complex, often incorporating an eclectic mix of talented staff, personalized treatment combinations, and ongoing modifications of programs, it may be best to measure fidelity through multiple approaches to collect the best and most reliable information. Program architects and researchers must identify the critical components of an approach and distill those that are essential and nonessential to program integrity. In their review of the literature on fidelity measurement, Bond and his colleagues (2000) recommended a mix of chart reviews, observations of team meetings, surveys of clients and staff, interviews with staff, and fidelity checklists or scales. Such a multimodal approach—which can include both quantitative and qualitative measures—is more likely to accurately capture the full range of implementation.

Development of a fidelity measurement procedure may take time and resources, but the effort is rewarded because these measures ensure consistency across programs. One of the most frequently cited examples of a fidelity index in the clinical literature is the Assertive Community Treatment (ACT) scale, which was based on expert ratings and the literature to reflect critical dimensions of the program (McGrew, Bond, & Dietzen, 1994; Teague, Drake, & Ackerman, 1995).

Kaskutas, Greenfield, Borkman, and Room (1998) created a Social Model Philosophy Scale to examine the extent to which an alcohol treatment program follows a social model approach to treatment. This scale contains 33 questions divided into six conceptual domains that cover physical environment, staff role, authority base, view of substance abuse problems, governance, and community orientation (Kaskutas et al., 1998). This type of instrument could be developed for all the major treatment philosophies, such as therapeutic communities, cognitive behavioral programs, and so on, to determine adherence to the main principles of the treatment approach.

In his review of program fidelity measurement, Orwin (2000) emphasized the importance of including an assessment of context. Programs function within a broad community context, and these contextual elements may play a part in determining program outcomes. For example, a program that is implementing an evidence-based treatment approach is affected by the wider array of services that are available—or unavailable—in a given community. Measures often used to study context include:

- Analysis of social and health indicators based on publicly available data from census, state, or municipal sources.
- Surveys of available local health and social services, including residential treatment beds available, housing programs, and job training services.
- Interviews with agency personnel about the availability and quality of local social and health services.
- Surveys that measure the collaboration that exists between and among local service providers.

Understanding how thoroughly an evidence-based program was implemented may be key to explaining outcomes, maintaining program quality, and contributing to the treatment field's overall understanding of what works, when it works, and why it works. There is another advantage to assessing fidelity through process evaluation. Key barriers to successful implementation sometimes can be identified and then corrected.

Outcome Evaluation

Outcome evaluations have typically focused on reductions in levels of alcohol or drug use and abstinence as the primary dependent variables. While these variables are extremely useful in understanding whether or not treatments are effective, there are other outcomes that may tell us even more about how treatments work over time. For example, it may be relevant to tease out more detail, such as the length of time of a relapse episode, number of relapses in a given time frame, events surrounding an instance of relapse (triggers), time period between treatment and relapse, and whether reduction in use led to abstinence. Moreover, programs may be interested in observing *mediating* or *short-term* outcomes, that is, early indicators that may be related to treatment success or failure, such as employment, family stability, mental and physical health, life satisfaction, degree of client motivation, and number of arrests. Depending on the program and the population, these indicators (separately or in combination) may be theoretically related to whether or not and how a client changes substance use patterns.

It is important for program staff and evaluators to untangle this complex mix of interventions, environmental context, mediating indicators, and outcomes. It may be helpful to articulate a "theory of change" in the context of a logic model that describes how the treatment program's activities result in measurable outcomes. Logic models are also very important in developing a process evaluation, although they may be less relevant for assessing program fidelity.

The Center for Substance Abuse Treatment (CSAT) proposed the use of a logic model that can provide a linkage between treatment and evaluation activities, ultimately supporting service improvement (Devine, 1999). A logic model states a clear path from etiology to treatment design to expected outcomes. CSAT describes a logic model as consisting of four parts:

1. *Conditions and context*—description of the context in which the treatment program operates, including target population characteristics, community characteristics and resources, and government and health care system policies related to treatment services.

2. *Activities*—services that make up the treatment program.

3. *Short-term outcomes*—proxy or mediating outcomes that are expected to result following or in the course of treatment, such as reduced use of alcohol or retention in treatment.

4. *Long-term outcomes*—often called impacts or goals, these outcomes may include such goals as family reunification. (Devine, 1999)

Other models, including the approach for developing logic models created by the Centers for Disease Control and Prevention (CDC) and the United Way, offer slightly varying components, such as stating inputs (e.g., resources and staffing) and outputs (e.g., treatment plan) (Centers for Disease Control and Prevention, 1999; United Way of America, 1996). Models can be drawn using boxes and arrows or as matrices, as shown in Table 5.1. Many authors recommend creating an outcome logic model that starts with research questions to focus the model and includes indicators and data sources. The simplified example in Table 5.1 integrates these approaches using the example of an alcohol treatment program.

Table 5.1 Sample Outcome Logic Model

Research Question	Activities	Short-Term Outcomes	Short-Term Indicators and Data Sources	Long-Term Outcomes	Long-Term Indicators and Data Sources
1. Did services result in a long-term change in drinking behavior and improved health and social functioning?	1. Motivational interviews with trained counselor	1. Expressed motivation to change behavior	1. Evidence of readiness to change based on scale scores or therapist report	1. Long-term change in use patterns (3-month, 6-month, past year)	1. Change in self-reported alcohol use, frequency and quantity
		2. Change in recent (1-week, 30-day) use of alcohol	2. & 3. Change in self-reported alcohol use, frequency and quantity	2. Family relationships	2. Change in nature of family relationships (interview, family functioning scale score)
		3. Change in quantity of alcohol consumed in past week/month		3. Employment	3. Job initiation and continuation
		4. Change in depression symptoms (or other mental health indicator)	4. CES-D or Beck Depression Inventory	4. Mental health improvement	4. CES-D or Beck Depression Inventory

This logic model helps demonstrate that there may be more than one way to measure any outcome—the indicators and data sources may give different information—self-reports, changes on mental health checklists, counselor reports about client motivation, and so on.

Owen (2003) provides a step-by-step guide for the measurement of client outcomes. Some of the highlights of this book are noted below, in the form of questions to guide the selection of outcome measurement tools or systems. Readers are encouraged to consult Owen's book for more detail on this important issue of measuring outcomes.

Who Wants to Know? Different stakeholders are interested in different kinds of outcomes. For example, a licensing or accrediting board will ask for different information than the managed care payers or advisory board members. Others who may ask for outcome data may include referral agencies, clients and/or their families, criminal justice agencies, administrators of the agency in which the program resides, and individual counselors in the program who want to know how their clients do.

What Do They Want to Know? Again, different stakeholders have differing needs for outcome data. A Department of Health and Human Services (DHHS) referral source may want to know if the treatment program produces better parents, a criminal justice agency might want to know about the impact of treatment on recidivism rates, and advisory board members might want to know how many clients are abstinent at the end of treatment and how long they stay that way. Since most agencies must answer to many stakeholders, the outcome measurements must be broad enough to cover these diverse needs. Some examples of outcomes that are often measured in substance abuse treatment programs include:

- Alcohol and drug use outcomes: type, quantity, frequency, whether client meets some diagnostic criteria.
- Treatment outcomes: retention rates, treatment graduation rates, average number of days in treatment, participation in self-help groups, treatment motivation.
- Mental health outcomes: current symptoms and diagnoses, changes in mental health status, stability of mental health conditions, use of mental health services.
- Physical health outcomes: rates of diseases related to substance abuse, current symptoms, use of physical health care services.
- Quality-of-life outcomes: education, employment, job satisfaction, independent living, housing, and so on.
- Legal issues: involvement in the criminal justice system.

- Family and relationship issues: significant other, children, family of origin.
- Cultural issues: identification with and support of a peer network or social group; cultural values and recovery.
- Spiritual issues: identification of and attention to spiritual needs in treatment and recovery; use of spiritual resources.

How Will You Define Your Outcome Variables? Think of the outcomes listed above. There are multiple ways to define and measure each one. For example, if abstinence is the major outcome variable, how is abstinence defined? From all substances or just from the drug of choice? By the end of the active treatment phase or 6 months later? Continuous abstinence or number of abstinent days between lapses? How will it be measured—self-report or a more objective measure such as urinalysis (UA) or blood test? What is the difference between a lapse and a relapse?

How and When Will Outcome Data Be Collected? Who will collect outcome data? Data can be collected as structured client interviews, self-administered surveys, follow-up phone calls, chart or record reviews, or some combination of these. Will data be collected by the counseling staff, clerical staff, or a research assistant, and how will this affect the data collection (e.g., could counselors have more investment in certain kinds of outcomes, or will clients report more honestly to a former counselor versus an independent data collector)?

Program Evaluation

Program evaluation is often a combination of client outcome and process evaluation, and is necessary to guide the further development of an agency. Program evaluation is sometimes considered the "ugly stepsister" of research. Academic researchers often think of it as "soft science" or too time-consuming and messy, so they do not get involved. Treatment providers think of evaluation as a necessary evil that eats up their budget. Policymakers require program evaluation information for accountability's sake, but often do not provide much guidance in doing evaluation. Is there a way to bring evaluation into a practice-research collaboration that will be more mutually beneficial to stakeholders? Many fields are exploring the use of empowerment evaluation.

> Empowerment evaluation is an evaluation approach that aims to increase the likelihood that programs will achieve results by increasing the capacity of program stakeholders to plan, implement, and evaluate their own programs. (Fetterman & Wandersman, 2005, p. 27)

The core principles of empowerment evaluation are quite compatible with the evidence-based practice movement and include the following:

1. Improvement of services

2. Community ownership of evaluation data (rather than the evaluator owning the data)

3. Inclusion (all stakeholders in a community are included in the process)

4. Democratic participation (requires "authentic collaboration" and transparency)

5. Social justice (committed to fair and equitable allocation of resources and services; evaluation is a tool to identify and rectify disparities)

6. Community knowledge (members of a community are experts on their own groups, recognizing that lived experience is a valid form of knowledge, equal to science-generated knowledge)

7. Evidence-based strategies (empirical science is important, but should be adopted with caution and in accordance with local context and community norms)

8. Capacity-building (empowerment evaluation provides skills to stakeholders that increase their capacity to improve circumstances in their communities)

9. Organizational learning (the process requires an openness to change, continual striving for improvement and systems thinking and promotes problem-solving skills)

10. Accountability (heightens an agency's or community's sense of responsibility to the public and its specific stakeholders, as well as accountability to the agency itself; accountability becomes self-driven rather than other-driven)

Conclusions

In conclusion, integrating fidelity assessments and traditional process evaluation with outcome evaluations can supply critical information about what really works in bringing about sustained improvements for all types of clients. Outcome measurement is time-consuming and expensive, but ultimately necessary to the survival of an agency.

6

A Research Primer

Overview, Hypotheses, and Variables

For many substance abuse counselors, executive directors, and policy-makers without research backgrounds, the idea of research is mysterious and daunting—research reports in the form of journal articles are difficult to read and full of statistical jargon, the results are confusing and contradictory, or they make no sense in the reality of clinical experience. Some people were required to take a research design or statistics course in their training programs, but they were often too esoteric to apply directly to clinical work. Many people in the substance abuse treatment field have had no research training at all, but are expected to participate in research data collection, to keep current with research findings, to evaluate their own programs or agencies, and/or to decide how to implement evidence-based practices at their agencies. The next four chapters provide a primer for people who have never taken a research course, and a brief review for those who have. All examples are drawn from the substance abuse field, and the chapters cover the "nuts and bolts" of research methods without a great deal of detail about the statistical procedures. There is little statistical jargon in this chapter, although there are definitions of statistical terms for those who want that information.

Why Is Research Important?

Success with the evidence-based practice movement hinges on developing research-savvy leaders in the substance abuse treatment field. Research related to substance abuse treatment is relatively new, and many research studies suffer from major limitations and flaws. A research-savvy provider will be able to detect the limitations. Thus far, no one has established clear, widely accepted guidelines for determining what constitutes an evidence-based practice. Research-informed treatment providers need to be part of the process for determining those guidelines (along with clinically informed researchers). The purpose of this chapter is to help leaders in the field to develop critical skills for evaluating the research in substance abuse treatment.

The reality is that everyone engages in research all the time without thinking about it. Every time a staff member asks, "Why is this client so resistant?" and tries to figure out an answer, that is a form of research. The only difference between daily problem-solving activities and what gets reported in a research journal is how systematic the process was. If the staff member carefully considered the theoretical reasons for resistance, developed a method to reduce the resistance, tried it out on the client, and gathered some kind of measure of resistance before and after trying the method, that would be called single-subject case research (or what some, including Scott Miller, have called "practice-based evidence"). If what was learned with one client was extended to other clients, and evaluated, that is even closer to empirical research methods.

Being research-savvy could benefit individuals personally in their jobs, enhancing their ability to interpret research articles and pull out significant findings that could inform clinical practice. This knowledge will also make grant writing easier, aid in the development of needs assessments or outcome measurement systems for an agency, and/or facilitate collaborating on research projects that are conducted onsite.

This chapter focuses on one particular kind of research—applied quantitative studies in clinical settings that potentially can inform clinical practice. Lab research on animals, human tissues, and/or brain scans can provide valuable information about the etiology and potential treatments of substance abuse in the long run, but rarely have any immediate application to the field, so these will not be used as examples here. Qualitative research will be explored in more detail in Chapter 9.

Types of Research

Quantitative and Qualitative

Chapters 6 through 8 focus on quantitative research, since most guidelines for evidence-based practice are based on the presence of empirical research support. Quantitative methods were derived from the natural sciences and constitute the "scientific method." In the scientific method, objective data, detectable by our senses (empirical data), are gathered and subjected to statistical analyses. In contrast, qualitative research is not concerned with being objective. Indeed, its focus is on finding out what people perceive to be true or right, not what is actually true. If a researcher wants to know how people make sense of their experiences, rather than count or classify their experiences, qualitative research is more helpful. Table 6.1 compares quantitative and qualitative methods. Both types of research are important in the generation of knowledge, but quantitative methods have been privileged in Western science, and are more useful in determining which practices produce better outcomes.

Table 6.1   Comparison of Quantitative and Qualitative Methods

Quantitative	*Qualitative*
Objective—the researcher is detached and seeks to reduce as much bias as possible.	Subjective—the researcher is involved, and is one of the methods of the study.
Uses methods that count or classify.	Uses methods that identify subjective meanings and interpretations.
Uses a deductive process: start with theory and research questions and gather information to prove or disprove.	Uses an inductive process: gather information first to inform the development of theory and/or research questions.
Uses statistical analyses to determine if group differences or pre- and posttest measure differences are due to chance or not.	Focuses on identifying common themes in people's experiences.

Laboratory and Field Studies

Some research is done in strictly controlled laboratory settings in order to isolate the variables the researcher wants to study from all the background noise in the real world. However, lab settings are "ideal" and therefore not much like the real world. Most of the research reviewed in this book is done in the field. Field studies are messier, but more realistic and more likely to generalize across clinical settings. Before any new evidence-based practice is adopted, several studies must examine it in field settings.

The Research Process (Step by Step)

The research process is relatively simple. The first step is to come up with an idea or research question (sometimes called a hypothesis if it is in the form of a statement rather than a question), develop a method to answer the question, find some people to study, collect information from them, enter the data into a computer or other analytical tool and analyze it, and write a report or article. The next several sections go through each step of the process and outline some of the problems that can occur. Table 6.2 outlines the process, and gives an example of each step.

Research Questions/Hypotheses

Quality research hinges on the precision of the research questions. The hypotheses or research questions must be crystal clear and measurable, or the research may be meaningless. Here are some examples of critiques of research questions:

Is substance abuse treatment effective?

This is clearly an important question and at the heart of accountability efforts in the field. However, there are major problems with a broad research question like this. First, what is treatment? Treatment means different things to different people. Is it detoxification, inpatient, outpatient, or online treatment? What approach does treatment take—psychoanalytic, 12-step meetings, cognitive behavioral, aversive, pharmacological, or some eclectic combination of approaches? For what length of time: a week, a month, 3 months? Group or individual? For children, adolescents, young adults, middle-aged people, or older adults? For white, middle-class professionals or for homeless teens? Second, what do we mean by "effective"—abstinence,

Table 6.2   Steps in the Research Process

Step	Example
1. Identify a problem and pose it as a research question or hypothesis.	Women seem to drop out of the program more frequently and sooner than men. Staff notice that the women who drop out seem more anxious and "flighty." The agency poses this question: "Does the presence of anxiety disorders contribute to premature treatment dropout for women?"
2. Define the variables of interest.	Operational definitions will be needed for: Independent—anxiety disorder (how will it be defined and measured?) and gender. Dependent: Premature dropout (number of days in treatment? Did they complete the program?) Possible confounding variables: other differences in women that could account for premature dropout, such as childcare responsibilities; treatment program variables.
3. Decide who will be studied.	All clients starting treatment from June to September of this year.
4. Decide how they will be studied.	Anxiety disorder structured interview is included as part of intake assessments. A face-to-face interview that takes about 20 minutes to complete.
5. Decide when they will be studied.	Intake: Anxiety instrument Every 6 weeks: Review records and record who is still in treatment, and who has dropped out.
6. Collect data.	Intake counselor trained in anxiety assessment records the findings on client records along with demographic information (gender, age, ethnicity, education, substance use history, mental health history, and so on). Record the number of days in treatment and whether successfully completed treatment (yes or no).
7. Analyze data (the type of statistic selected is noted in parentheses).	Descriptive data to characterize the sample (e.g., 102 women and 267 men followed over the treatment period, mean age of 32, 68 percent stimulant users). Inferential statistics

(Continued)

Table 6.2   (Continued)

Step	Example
	to determine if there was a difference by gender and/or anxiety disorder.
	Presence of anxiety disorder:
	Men: 28 percent
	Women: 57 percent (chi square)
	Presence of PTSD:
	Men: 15 percent
	Women: 48 percent (chi square)
	Average # Days in Tx:
	Men: 62
	Women: 54 (t test)
	Gender by PTSD Diagnosis: percentage who drop out of treatment:
	Men with PTSD: 31 percent
	Men without PTSD: 35 percent
	Women with PTSD: 64 percent
	Women without: 32 percent
8. Interpret the results.	Think of all possible explanations for the findings—how many can be ruled out? It appears that PTSD, and not anxiety disorders in general, predicts the dropout rate for women. PTSD rate does not predict dropout rate for men.
9. Disseminate the findings.	Discuss in staff meetings. Write a report for board of directors or funders. Write an article about it. Make a poster to display at conferences.
10. The often-missing next step: Now what?	Train staff in anxiety disorders, particularly PTSD; continue to track dropout rates to see if training has an effect; refer clients for trauma interventions and/or treatment for anxiety.

reduction in use, fewer lost work days, a lower recidivism rate, or a happier spouse? Finally, what is "substance abuse"? Does that mean *Diagnostic and Statistical Manual of Mental Disorders, Fourth Edition* (DSM-IV) criteria or something else? Dependence on, or abuse of, alcohol, cocaine, nicotine, gambling, or food? A more precise research question might look something like the following:

Does an 8-week cognitive behavioral program for adolescent females in residential treatment reduce the use of drugs and alcohol over a 6-month period?

Even though this question is more specific, the researcher would need to elaborate on each of the terms in the question. How many hours of actual intervention are involved: an hour a day for 8 weeks, or 6 hours per day? What kinds of skills or knowledge does the program attempt to provide? How are "adolescent females" defined? Are they age 12, age 16, or a wide age range? What other characteristics of the sample are important: Are they urban or rural youth, racially mixed or all the same race, in school or dropouts, and so on. What is meant by "reduce" alcohol and drug use? How much of a reduction is sufficient to declare the program a success? When all these questions are answered, "operational definitions" have been established for the study.

Here is a research question that raises different kinds of issues:

Do women benefit more from Alcoholics Anonymous (AA) than men?

This is a very common type of research question, and it assumes that there are some clearly defined categories called man and woman. In reality, there are huge differences within any social category based on human characteristics such as race and ethnicity, age, gender, sexual orientation, socio economic status, religion, disability, and hundreds of other human differences. A question that pits women against men often denies the complexity of human existence and lumps all women into one category and all men into another. What if the client was born male, but underwent hormonal and surgical treatments at age 45 and now lives as a woman? What sex or gender is this client? The same problems arise with any large social grouping category, such as race or age. Not all Asian Americans are alike, nor are all Catholics, or all elderly women, or even all Latino urban youth. This does not mean that it is inappropriate to compare people based on these social categories; it just means that researchers consider the possibility that any difference they see might be due to something else entirely.

The discussion so far illustrates that the categories or words we use in everyday life are often vague or too simplistic to be suitable for research purposes. Because of the sloppiness of language, the researcher must carefully define all the variables of importance in a research study. This may seem like nitpicking, but the success of the entire study depends on the precision of the research questions and clear definition of the key variables.

Variables

There are several different kinds of variables used in research, and it is important to understand the differences among them. Here are some definitions:

- *Variable:* a factor that is measured, manipulated, or controlled in a research study.
- *Independent variables:* the variables that are studied or manipulated to determine their effect on an outcome. If clients are assigned to a coping skills group, or to treatment as usual, the type of treatment is the independent variable.
- *Dependent variables:* the outcomes or end results of the study (they "depend" on effects of the independent variables). In the case of a coping skills group, the dependent variable might be an increase in use of healthy coping and a decrease in unhealthy coping skills.
- *Confounding variables:* these are the things that were not taken into account in designing the study, but that may have influenced the results. These are factors so closely tied to the independent variables that they are difficult to sort out. For example, extraneous treatment variables such as family support, being on probation, or having to drop regular urinalyses (UAs) may influence the outcome, but were not measured.
- *Mediating variables:* some factors do not directly cause an outcome to occur but, in combination with other factors, might influence the result. It may be difficult to predict that one or more variables might turn out to be mediators. For example, providing wraparound services (the independent variable) may increase attendance in treatment groups (the mediator variable), and thus increase abstinence rates (the dependent variable).

Here is an example to make these definitions more clear. The study involves assessing the effects of naltrexone on alcohol craving in women. The plan is to give half the women in an inpatient treatment program a 4-week trial of naltrexone and compare them to the other half, who will receive treatment as usual. Alcohol craving will be measured on a daily basis, using a 0-to-10 rating scale where 0 is equal to no alcohol craving at all, and 10 is very strong craving. In this case, naltrexone (yes or no) is the independent variable. Naltrexone can be manipulated by giving it to some women but not others, but things like sex, age, race, and class can only be controlled but not changed. This study controls for sex or gender by studying only women. The dependent variable is the rating of alcohol craving. Alcohol craving cannot be measured directly, so the researcher must rely on a self-report measure. On the day that the study is to begin, 30 women are in residence and 80 percent are mothers. Motherhood may be a confounding variable in this case, because being a mother may be a major treatment motivator and might affect the perception of craving. Or perhaps a flu epidemic hits the agency during week 3 of the study, and none of the women experiences alcohol craving for a week because they are too sick. Some confounding variables are Mother Nature's gift, but researchers try to anticipate as many of them as possible before attempting a research project. Motherhood could be anticipated, while the flu epidemic cannot.

Mediating variables are ones that influence some outcome, but are not completely a cause of some phenomenon. For example, there is mounting evidence that child sexual abuse by itself is not a direct risk factor for later substance abuse, but emotional distress that comes from the sexual abuse for some people is the mediating variable. Thus, child sexual abuse has an indirect effect on substance abuse through emotional distress processes.

Research questions or hypotheses are not always directly labeled as such in journal articles, but may be embedded in paragraphs about the purpose of the study. For example, an article by Longshore, Grills, Anglin, and Annon (1997) states:

> This study examined demographic factors, drug-problem severity indicators, and social and personal resources as correlates of desire for help among African American drug users with no prior experience in treatment . . . Andersens' (1968, 1995) model of health behavior served as a heuristic for selecting the factors to be tested. In that model, help-seeking is a function of predisposing factors such as ethnicity and problem severity as well as enabling factors such as income and social support. Our study tested several predisposing and enabling factors as correlates of desire for help. In particular we sought to "unpack" the construct of ethnicity by testing ethnicity-related attitudes, perceptions, and experiences as predisposing factors potentially important to desire for help among African Americans. (pp. 755–756)

To translate, the research question could be paraphrased as "What is the role of ethnicity in help-seeking behavior for African American substance abusers?" Unfortunately, a somewhat convoluted, impersonal style of writing is required in most academic journals, making it difficult to pin down the precise purpose of the study. Some researchers write in a formal academic language that is frustrating for clinicians.

Conclusions

Creating good research questions is important, whether planning an experimental research study or designing a program evaluation. The following questions may be helpful in guiding the process of writing research questions.

- Are the terms clearly defined?
- Is the focus narrow enough to be accomplished?
- Can the chosen variables be accurately measured?
- Can the research question be answered directly, with information that is easy to obtain?
- Does it pass the "so what" test? Is the research of high priority? Will the information obtained by the study or evaluation be useful in some way?

7

Research Methods

This chapter addresses three critical steps in the research process. The first issue is related to procedures or research design, whether it is an experimental study or non-experimental. The second includes all the issues surrounding sample selection, such as issues of generalizability, representativeness, and human subjects concerns. The final issue addresses the many different methods for collecting data. The chapter will begin with a brief overview of the two major types of quantitative research designs: experimental and non-experimental. The type of design will influence the way the researcher goes about selecting a sample.

Two Basic Types of Research Designs

Is the goal of the study to examine something that is already present and has not yet been well described, or to manipulate or change some variable and see what happens? Experimental research manipulates variables to see what happens to the outcomes, whereas non-experimental research (sometimes referred to as descriptive or correlational research) involves no manipulation by the researcher. Table 7.1 compares and contrasts experimental and non-experimental research.

Non-experimental research is used to collect information about a problem or about a group of people and could include studies that:

- Look at the age of onset of use of certain drugs
- Count the number of senior citizens who report at least one alcohol-related problem

Table 7.1   Experimental and Non-Experimental Research

	Experimental Research	*Non-Experimental Research*
Purpose	To study what happens to an outcome when one factor is controlled or manipulated.	To study a phenomenon already there, or something that cannot be manipulated by the researcher.
Key Features	1. Random assignment of subjects to conditions. 2. A manipulation or intervention occurs. 3. There is a control or comparison group that does not get the intervention (or gets treatment as usual).	Can have some of these features, but not all.

- Assess the training needs of substance abuse counselors
- Examine the potential relationship between media and adolescent drug use
- Determine the percentage of alcoholics who develop liver disease

Non-experimental research can be cross-sectional or longitudinal. For example, in a longitudinal study, one could enlist a group of college students in their first year and follow them for the next 10 years to see what happens to their alcohol and drug use patterns. Descriptive research can use any data collection method, such as anonymous surveys, structured interviews, direct observations, or neuropsychological assessment. Descriptive studies only provide information about relationships among variables and cannot address cause-and-effect questions. For example, if a researcher collects information about adults who came from divorced families and finds that more of the adults of divorce smoke than expected, this does not mean that divorce causes smoking. Maybe some third factor causes both divorce and smoking.

Addressing cause-and-effect questions requires experimental research done over time. Experimental research has two main components: First, the researcher controls or manipulates some variables (the independent variables) to determine what will happen to other variables (the dependent or outcome variables). Second, there is a control or comparison group that does not get the manipulation or gets a different type of treatment. True experimental studies have a third requirement: random assignment of individuals to the conditions.

If data were collected on two groups of adults—those who experienced divorce in childhood (experimental group) and those who did not (comparison group)—and the divorce group contained more smokers, the researcher could not say that divorce caused smoking, but could be more sure of some sort of a relationship because of the difference between the divorce group and a comparison group. However, it is not an experimental study, because no variables were manipulated; the researcher only studied something already there (divorce), and there was no random assignment of subjects to group. If the researcher collected information on children at the time they were experiencing a divorce and followed them over the next 10 years and still found higher rates of smoking, he or she could still say only that there was a relationship between divorce and smoking. Divorce itself may not be a direct cause—perhaps children who have less adult supervision are more likely to start smoking, and children from divorced families are more likely to experience less adult supervision (an example of a mediating variable). Other factors in the child's home life, also associated with divorce, might contribute to smoking. For example, divorced parents may be more likely to smoke than intact parents, so the child grows up with smoking parents as role models. In this case of divorce and smoking, the researcher did not manipulate any variables, but controlled for the presence of divorce. It would be unethical to cause a divorce to see what happened to the children. While it would be more powerful to follow the individuals from childhood to adulthood, the study does not meet the criteria for an experimental study.

In the more classic experiment, there is some manipulation of variables. One agency decides to study the effects of vitamin therapy on cognitive functioning in individuals recovering from alcohol dependence on an inpatient unit. Patients are randomly assigned to one of three conditions. There are 45 residents, so 15 people are assigned to each of three groups:

Group 1: Multiple vitamin therapy—Recommended Daily Allowance (RDA)

Group 2: Multiple vitamins plus extra B complex vitamins

Group 3: No vitamins

Before starting to administer the vitamins to some clients, researchers could measure cognitive functioning by some kind of neuropsychological measure such as memory, attention, or abstract reasoning, or perhaps they would ask the staff to rate each client on some cognitive dimension. Then the intervention begins. Depending on the length of the intervention, follow-up assessments could be scheduled at 1 month, 2 months, 6 months, and 1 year, or they could collect regular measurements daily or weekly. The researcher might expect to see improvements in cognitive functioning the longer the client is clean and sober, but if the vitamin therapy works, the vitamin groups should improve faster than the control group. The sooner their cognitive functioning improves, the sooner they can benefit from therapy, so this kind of research could have very practical applications. The researcher had a measure of cognitive function that resulted in a number from 0 (severely impaired cognition) to 10 (normal cognitive functioning). Table 7.2 shows some fictitious results of the study.

The statistical analysis suggests that the groups are no different at baseline or at 4 weeks, but by 8 and 12 weeks, the vitamin groups are showing much better cognitive functioning than the control group. Overall, the multivitamin plus B vitamin group showed the greatest net gain in cognitive functioning, increasing by 3.8 units compared to the RDA vitamin group, which improved by 3.2 units, and the control group, which improved by only 2.9 units. If there was no control group, the researcher would not have a measure of "normal" cognitive improvement over time due solely to detoxification from drugs and alcohol. Control groups are essential in experimental research.

Research, whether experimental or descriptive, can be done in a laboratory where the researcher has greater control over many variables, but which removes the client from "real life." Field studies are more like real life, but are harder to control. The vitamin study is a good example. In a controlled laboratory setting, all meal preparation and snacks could be controlled to isolate the influence of vitamins on the outcomes. In real life, some clients may get a much higher dose of vitamins just through the foods that they choose compared to other clients. If the treatment assignment was random, the researcher can assume that these other factors will balance out across the groups. In the case of the assessments, the lab setting could provide much more control over conditions: every client could be given the neuropsychological assessments in the same soundproof room with no window by the same researcher. In a field study, assessments are often arranged

Table 7.2   Effects of Vitamin Therapy on Cognitive Functioning

Grp	Baseline	Vitamins	4 wks	8 wks	12 wks
1	4.2	Yes	4.6	6.5	7.4
2	3.9	Yes	4.8	6.8	7.7
3	4.3	No	4.6	5.1	6.2

around the agency schedule, with some done in private rooms and others in the cafeteria between meals! It is much harder to control for noise level, interruptions, and many other distractions in the field setting. Clinical agencies are notoriously unpredictable sites for data collection, and poor performance on a memory test could be due to the person yelling in the next room.

The Gold Standard: Randomized Clinical Trials

This book focuses on evidence-based practice models, thus on research related to treatment effectiveness rather than prevalence studies. Randomized clinical trials (RCTs) are considered the best way to study treatment approaches. RCTs use clinical samples instead of a general population sample. In a clinical trial, the population might be all the adult clients in an inpatient program. In order for the study to be a randomized clinical trial, every client entering the program during the study period must have the same chance of being selected for the intervention, such as a new program or a trial medication. The others get the standard treatment. Unlike "true" clinical trials, in which a control group gets no treatment and the experimental group gets a treatment, in a substance abuse treatment center, it is considered unethical to assign a client to a no-treatment control group. Subject assignment to groups can become a problem if a staff member decides that one of the treatments might be better than the other and biases the treatment selection by assigning his or her clients to one of the treatments. Usually this is done with the best of intentions, as the staff member is choosing what she or he believes to be the best option for that client.

An example of subject selection for a clinical trials type of research might include the following description:

> Subjects were drawn from the outpatient admissions to 10 large substance abuse treatment agencies (4 East Coast, 4 West Coast, 2 Midwestern) from January 1, 2000 to March 31, 2000. Subjects were randomly assigned to (A) the regular treatment programs of the agency, all of which were 12-step-based programs with primarily group therapies; or (B) an individually administered cognitive behavioral program. A total of 2,000 participants (1,000 in 12-step treatment and 1,000 in cognitive behavioral treatment) will be assessed upon entry into the program, upon exit from the program, and at 6-month intervals for 2 years thereafter. The dependent measures will include amount of substance use (categorized as abstinence, reduced use from baseline, same amount of use as baseline, or greater use than baseline) and family and social adjustment.

Clinical trials projects vary in size and scope. Some are multi-site studies with large sample sizes; others are located in small treatment programs with 10 to 20 participants. They can be geographically diverse to broaden the scope of the population and to control for any differences that might occur in patterns of substance use or treatment approaches.

Other Research Designs

Randomized clinical trials are not always feasible, and most treatment approaches are studied with a range of research designs. Often, researchers begin with small pilot studies with no comparison or control groups, and collect data before and after the intervention, with limited follow-up data. Or a small study compares the new treatment approach to treatment as usual, using two different programs instead of random assignment of clients to avoid "contamination" of effects of the intervention. For example, suppose that adolescents in one residential treatment program are randomized into two groups: one gets an HIV risk reduction program and the other gets treatment as usual. Are the clients in the program likely to avoid talking to their peers about what they discuss in the intervention? The way to avoid this is to have the comparison group come from a different treatment program that is as much like the one where the intervention is delivered as possible. This is a quasi-experimental study.

Selecting a Sample

Once the research design has been selected and the research questions and variables are as precise, objective, and replicable as possible, the next step is to identify a sample, or a group of people to study. It is never possible to study the entire population of interest—for example, all methamphetamine users—so methods of selecting a sample that represent the population or some subset of the population are used. If the research question calls for determining the prevalence or frequency of some problem, such as the percent of methamphetamine users who experience heart failure, a random sample is the most desirable. This is because nonrandom samples are often biased in some way. If the sample was identified through an emergency room, there would be more people with heart failure than if the data were collected at Narcotics Anonymous (NA) meetings. For a truly representative, random sample, every person in the population must have an equal chance of being selected. If the state of Iowa wanted to collect information on the need for treatment for methamphetamine, how could they go about identifying who needs treatment?

There are multiple sampling procedures that could be used, but each one has some drawbacks. Most random population studies use one or more of the following methods:

- *Random digit dialing procedures.* In this method, the researchers would get a random sample from all the phone numbers for the state of Iowa, screen them to find only personal residences, and then interview people by phone. This method excludes people who do not have phones, who do not answer their phones, or who are rarely home. Are any of these true of methamphetamine users?
- *Census address data.* Some studies use the last census data to identify people and draw a random sample from those addresses (such as using a random numbers table to select addresses). Census data have a number of problems, too. Obviously, it does not capture people who are homeless—either without housing at all or in transitory housing with others. And it is influenced by the length of time between the most recent census and the study. If the study were done in April 2005, the researchers might only have access to 2000 census data. How many people might have moved in that 5-year span, particularly among a drug-using population? Even if the researchers found people at home for in-home interviews, are drug users more or less likely to agree to be in a research study than non-drug users? Using addresses, the researcher might mail out a survey—how many people take the time to complete a survey that comes in the mail?
- *Driver's license data.* Most adults in Iowa drive cars, so a study could draw a random sample from driver's license data. This would miss people who do not drive, who have had their licenses revoked, or who check the confidentiality box on the application form for a driver's license. Are any of these likely for substance abusers?
- *House-to-house selection.* Researchers could randomly select several geographic regions in the state, representative of the urban and rural mix, and then draw maps of target neighborhoods. A door-to-door interviewer could knock on people's doors and survey them. This, like the census approach, misses those who are homeless, and relies on catching people at home. It might also produce unintended bias if the cities or regions selected are highly segregated by ethnicity, which many parts of the United States are. It is also the most labor- and time-intensive method (and therefore very expensive). So instead of going to people's homes, some researchers choose locations where many people congregate and collect data there. However, selection of the location is very important. A booth at an upscale mall identifies a very different type of respondent than a table at the local Women, Infants and Children (WIC) office.

A lot of these methods require considerable time and effort and very large numbers of subjects to answer the research questions. For example, if methamphetamine users make up 1 percent of the Iowa population and research shows that about 1 percent of methamphetamine users have heart failure, the researcher might need to survey more than 10,000 people just to find one methamphetamine user with heart failure.

Random population studies are important for collecting prevalence or frequency data, because clinical samples are not always typical of "the substance abuser." Clinicians who work in treatment programs see only a small segment of the substance-abusing population (the 10 percent or so who get treatment), and the people who seek treatment or get court-ordered to treatment are probably different in significant ways from the substance abuser who gets help only from Alcoholics Anonymous (AA), Narcotics Anonymous (NA), or a health care provider or who gets better without any professional help at all.

Much of the research in the substance abuse treatment field uses convenience samples rather than random population samples. If the research question is exploratory or if some preliminary information about something is needed, convenience samples are cheaper and easier to get. Instead of doing a random population study of effects of methamphetamine on the heart, a health screening of all methamphetamine users in 10 substance abuse treatment agencies in Iowa might provide a preliminary answer. The researchers would have to say that the results may not generalize to methamphetamine users who do not get treatment, but at least could make some conclusions about the treatment population.

Generalizability of Samples

One of the most important things to consider when reviewing research publications about evidence-based practices is to determine if the sample studied is comparable to the clients in the agency considering changing to the new practice. If an agency is searching for help on a treatment approach for pregnant female cocaine addicts, then a random population study might not be helpful. Neither would a VA hospital study of male Vietnam War veterans with cocaine addiction. If the agency is in a predominantly white, rural community, research on an urban sample of mostly African American women might not be so helpful, either. It may be difficult to find a study with a sample that exactly matches the agency needs, but new practices must be implemented with caution when the sample is too different.

The following example illustrates another point. A research study about older adults living in two retirement communities in one Northeastern town finds heavy drinking patterns in 30 percent of the men and 22 percent of the women. In 5 years at a substance abuse treatment agency in the same town, the executive director reports, it has never had a client over the age of 60. How does one reconcile this difference between the research finding and clinical experience? There may be a tendency to reject the research finding without considering possible reasons for the discrepancy.

"Heavy drinking" can be defined in different ways. Perhaps none of the people in this sample who were "heavy drinkers" based on a measure of alcohol consumption had experienced any alcohol-related problems, and that is why the agency had never seen adults of this age. Perhaps a measure of consumption is not the same as meeting *Diagnostic and Statistical Manual of Mental Disorders* (DSM) criteria. Or maybe this sample was unusual in some way—perhaps these two retirement centers had recreational activities that regularly included alcohol (such as weekly bus trips to a riverboat casino) and these older adults were not representative of the older population of the town or county. Or perhaps the community or the treatment agency does not do a very good job of identifying substance abuse in this population. Another reason for the disparity might be due to attitudes: perhaps older adults perceive (rightly) that they would not fit in well in a typical substance abuse treatment program, and that the younger clients and staff might not understand their issues. This is a good example where clinical experience can help explain research findings. If researchers and treatment providers had worked together to design the study and interpret the results, the study may have been more useful.

Here is a verbatim quotation from an article about an HIV risk reduction intervention program for women. The authors describe their sample as follows:

One hundred seventeen (n = 117) women were recruited into the intervention following admission into a publicly funded inpatient chemical dependence treatment facility. Average stay in the program was 42 days. Thirteen women were discharged early or irregularly, leaving 104 women eligible to complete the intervention. The mean age of the sample was 34.2 (SD = 8.0) and mean years of education was 11.4 (SD = 2.3). Forty-three percent (43.4%) of the women were African American, 54.8% were white, and 1.9% were Native American. Most (86.5%) were unemployed at the time of admission [more detail on employment, children, income, and relationships was provided here] . . . Voluntary HIV testing was offered to the women on admission and 89.4% reported being tested upon admission. . . . Over one-quarter (27.2%) reported self-injection with needle sharing since 1979 and 52.9% reported a lifetime STD. Mean number of lifetime sex partners was 86.2 (SD = 181, median 27.5). (Eldridge et al., 1997, p. 65)

This description provides enough detail to determine if the sample is comparable to any given treatment program. If it is similar, staff may expect the intervention to work in their agency as well. Even though it can be somewhat tedious to read all these numbers, they really are important. Sometimes there are interesting or unexpected findings in these descriptions of the sample. What about the mean number of sexual partners? This finding will be used as an example when discussing data analysis in Chapter 8. Is it unusual for a group of women to report an average of 86 sexual partners in their lifetimes?

Another issue has to do with sample size. How many people must be studied to make the study a "good" one? This question has no real answer, but there are some guidelines to consider. If the study is an exploratory study or deals with a rare population, even a study with only a few people in it could be useful. For example, at the beginning of the methamphetamine epidemic, there were some qualitative studies of women users, asking them to compare methamphetamine use to other drugs and to talk about the reasons that they used methamphetamine. Some of these studies had only 20 to 30 participants, but they gave us some ideas about the attraction of meth for women. However, if the research is concerned with testing a new treatment approach or determining if one program works better than another, then the more participants the better. It would not be ethical or responsible to recommend some medication for clients if it had been tested only on 100 adult men of ages 19 to 25.

Even though, in general, the more participants the better, studies with very large sample sizes, such as studies of more than 1,000 people, carry another risk. The larger the sample size, the more likely it is to find statistically significant differences among groups. This can be good if the differences are meaningful. If studying how many men and women report loneliness on a scale of 0 (not lonely at all) to 100 (extremely lonely) and the sample is large enough, even a trivial difference might be found to be statistically significant. In this hypothetical case, the men report a mean score of 85.4 and the women report a mean loneliness score of 84.8. This difference would have no practical application whatsoever.

There is one last issue to address about sampling. That is the ethical issue of consent versus informed consent. At one time, it was believed that it was enough for potential participants to say "yes," they would participate in research. Now the legal and ethical rights of potential participants to know exactly what they are saying yes to are recognized. That is, researchers must provide full disclosure of what participation in the study involves: how much time is involved, what kind of procedures will be done, are there any risks to the participant, are there are any benefits, are they going to be given any incentives for participating, how will participant confidentiality be ensured, and what will be done with the information? Informed consent is a sticky issue when it comes to people who have mental disabilities, who are under legal age, who are incarcerated or under the supervision of the criminal justice system, who are currently involved in illegal activities, or who might be under the influence of a substance when the consent form is signed. In general, researchers are ethically bound to protect the rights of participants in terms of confidentiality, dignity, and safety. Participants have the right to say no to a research project without affecting their care in any way, and even if they say "yes" and sign a consent form, they have the right to withdraw at any time. The next section describes the process that researchers must follow to get permission to do research with humans. (There are other procedures to ensure ethical conduct with animals.)

Institutional Review Boards

Over the years, there have been entirely too many horror stories about unethical research—giving subjects painful electric shocks just to see how they handle stress, withholding treatment to study the "natural history" of some disease, using prisoners to test potentially dangerous experimental drugs, and so on. Because not all researchers are born with the ethical conduct gene, all research must be reviewed and approved by an Institutional Review Board (IRB) or Human Subjects Review Committee. Every university has at least one of these committees, and sometimes large community agencies that engage in considerable research have their own. Members of IRBs include researchers, lawyers, practitioners, specialists in ethics, consumers, and community advocates. Their job is to protect the rights of people participating in research from unwarranted harm. For example, the harm that can come to participants in research studies can include consequences of loss of confidentiality, unacceptable risks, misrepresentation of risks, coercion, and/or lack of safeguards.

Loss of Confidentiality

How will the researcher protect the identity of the participant? Does the questionnaire contain items that pertain to illegal activities (e.g., Have you ever stolen money or goods to get drugs? Have you ever written bad checks intentionally?) How will the researcher avoid subpoena of these documents? What if a woman is hiding from an abusive spouse in a substance abuse treatment center? Is there anything in the research protocol that may jeopardize her safety? Obviously, the researcher would not want to send a questionnaire to that spouse to collect collateral information. The researcher must prepare a document that informs the participant of how confidentiality will be protected and under what circumstances confidentiality might be broken. In clinical practice, confidentiality is broken only in cases of potential harm to self or others, such as reports of child abuse or suicidal or homicidal thoughts—the same would apply for research studies. Confidentiality must be broken if clients pose a serious danger to themselves or others.

Risk-Benefit Analyses

The IRB must determine that the study has more benefits than risks to make it worthwhile to subjects. For example, if the study involves asking people entering a substance abuse treatment program to recall traumatic childhood events, such as sexual abuse, but does not offer any treatment or crisis intervention for them, the study may be deemed too risky. What if the medication that reduces alcohol craving has potentially dangerous side effects? What if one out of every 1,000 persons who take it has a stroke? Is that worth the risk? Maybe three out of every 1,000 alcoholics who do not take the drug will die from an automobile accident. IRBs are charged with making the determination of risk versus benefit.

Misrepresentation of Risks or Benefits

Sometimes researchers exaggerate the importance of their study or they minimize the risks—or do not consider what might be risky to another person. The consent forms and documents that inform subjects about the research must be accurate. If there is no immediate benefit to the subject, the forms must say so. If the treatment is experimental, no claims can be made about possible outcomes, even if the researcher is pretty sure that it will be beneficial. What about subjects who are assigned to control groups? They have no potential for added benefits at all, and must be informed of this.

Coercion

At all costs, coercion must be avoided. No individual must feel like she or he has to participate in a research study in order to avoid jail, to get better treatment, or even to make the substance abuse counselor happy. Clients who feel coerced into a study are less likely to be honest, may not comply with all aspects of the study, or may even try to sabotage the study.

Safeguards

The informed consent document must specify all the potential risks and how they will be dealt with. How will the researcher protect confidentiality, monitor the individual for adverse effects, avoid unnecessary intrusion into their lives, and so on?

Research Procedures/Data Collection

This section deals with the carrying out of research. There are a number of different methods of conducting research, which will be summarized under three categories below. The first is related to the timing of the data collection (cross-sectional versus longitudinal), the second has to do with how information is obtained (what kinds of measurement techniques are used), and the third is related to the independent variables. (Are researchers manipulating or changing something to determine its effect, or only studying something that is already present and waiting to be discovered?)

Cross-Sectional Versus Longitudinal Designs

Research designs are varied and depend on the research questions. If researchers want to estimate how many slots are needed for inpatient and outpatient treatment programs in a particular city or county, one kind of method—such as an anonymous survey or a phone interview sent to every home—might be helpful. This could be done at one point in time, a cross-sectional design. However, to study the effectiveness of massage therapy in reducing alcohol and drug use, the same people must be studied over time (longitudinal design). An anonymous survey would not work, because the people must be located at a later time and their responses from one time to another linked. Longitudinal research is much harder to do, because researchers have to be able to find people after they leave treatment and get full cooperation from them in completing follow-up measures. The attrition rate of longitudinal studies in the field of substance abuse is very high because substance abusers so often move, hide from authority figures, become incarcerated, die, are afraid to tell the truth, or just cannot be located. Even if located, some will have relapsed but will not want to reveal this information for various, usually good, reasons.

Cross-sectional research can offer information about the relationships among variables, but cannot answer cause-and-effect questions or discuss changes over time. Only certain kinds of longitudinal experimental research can address potential reasons for change. This is important to keep in mind. For example, a study that collected information about retrospective memories of childhood sexual abuse in people currently in substance abuse treatment found that 75 percent of the women and 40 percent of the men had experienced sexual abuse. This study cannot conclude that sexual abuse causes substance abuse, but only conclude that they often seem to go together. However, if the study began when the participants were children who were reported as experiencing sexual abuse or not, and the researcher found them again 10 to 15 years later and measured their alcohol and drug use, then the researcher could *possibly* address the natural course of post-sexual abuse and development of substance abuse. Remember that human behavior is extraordinarily complex, and that no study is likely to be able to assess all the variables that might be related to the development of substance abuse. It is difficult to definitively say that any one risk factor causes the other.

This next study describes a longitudinal design:

> We report here on changes in substance use over a 12 month period among a cohort of men recruited at a gay-identified outpatient substance abuse treatment agency in San Francisco. This article describes the treatment services available at the agency and the demographic characteristics of the men who seek services there, reports baseline levels of substance use and longitudinal changes in substance use over time and identifies predictors of different patterns of substance use at follow-up one year after entering treatment. (Paul, Barnett, Crosby, & Stall, 1996, p. 476)

Men were recruited into the study from April 1990 to October 1992 and included 321 men at baseline. They were given questionnaires to complete every 90 days. At the one-year follow-up, 261 men were still in the study, which is an excellent follow-up rate for this kind of study. Figure 7.1 is a simplified version of one of their graphs regarding the results for alcohol use patterns.

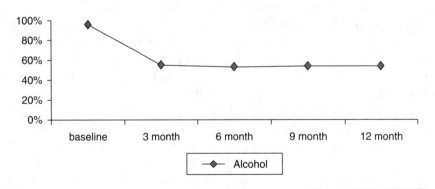

Figure 7.1   Paul et al. (1996) Data on Alcohol Use Patterns and Treatment

The results show that alcohol reductions for the group as a whole were dramatic in the first 3 months after entry into treatment, but leveled off after that. Almost all the men used alcohol at baseline (96 percent), but only 55 percent used any alcohol at 3 months. Because the study was longitudinal and followed the same men over time, the authors could investigate what was associated with alcohol reductions over time. They found that white men were less likely to reduce alcohol use than men of color, that men with more social problems at baseline were more likely to continue drinking, and that men with a "bar orientation" (who do most of their socializing in bars) did not reduce their drinking as much as men without a bar orientation.

Data Collection Methods

Research designs also vary in the methods by which data are collected. Information can be gathered from people in the following ways:

- Direct observation (watch what people actually do)
- Self-report measures (ask people what they think or know or ask them to perform some cognitive function). These measures can be in the form of structured interviews, open-ended interviews, IQ tests, neuropsychological measures, personality inventories, or paper and pencil questionnaires. These measures can be delivered face-to-face, via the computer, on the phone, or by mail-in questionnaires.
- Lab or physiological measures (blood tests, urine tests, x-rays, brain scans, etc.)
- Record reviews (gather information from hospital charts, arrest records, treatment records, newspaper stories, etc.)
- Collateral information (asking people who know the client about some aspect of their experience). Collateral sources could include spouses, children, parents, siblings, physicians, treatment counselors, probation officers, or social workers.

Each of these methods has advantages and disadvantages, and none is perfect. Direct observations are fine for measuring very objective and visible behaviors, such as the number of times a client interrupts someone in a group session. However, the observations are not helpful in understanding the motivation for the behavior or what the person might be thinking. In addition, just having an observer present may change people's behavior. Observational research can be done in one of two ways: non-participant observers would sit quietly in a corner and record their observations without intruding into the group. A participant observer would be involved in the group activity. For example, one researcher might go to Alcoholics Anonymous (AA) meetings and take notes without participating in any way, whereas another researcher could be a full participating member of the AA group and share experiences just like the other members. Would they get different kinds of information from the AA group? Might they interpret what happens in a group differently? How would informed consent issues need to be addressed differently for these two types of observational studies?

Self-report measures are often designed to address people's perceptions of motivation, thinking patterns, physical symptoms, or emotions, and are useful as long as the person is being honest, has sufficient cognitive skills to understand the question, and/or has adequate memory skills to recall past events accurately. In your experience, how are substance abusers at providing information about their drug use histories? Self-report measures can also be influenced by physical health. Compare the way clients feel 3 days after the last drink with the way they feel after 3 weeks—could there be differences in the way they think or feel, based just on degree of detoxification or stage of withdrawal? How often do researchers and clinicians try to collect information from someone who is still under the influence of a substance? Can researchers always tell who is under the influence? Sometimes researchers try to collect information from collateral sources to verify self-reports. For example, a sketchy history is obtained from a 39-year-old alcoholic man, so the researcher interviews his wife to verify his story, get more details, and get another perspective. What are the potential problems with his wife's history? Collateral sources are generally indirect and provide incomplete information and/or they are biased because of the perspective of the person who provides the collateral information.

Lab tests are often fairly objective, straightforward, and helpful in suggesting if a person has had a recent exposure to some drug or has tuberculosis or human immunodeficiency virus (HIV), but are not very helpful in planning a substance abuse treatment approach. Sometimes blood tests are inaccurate— a person who ate a poppy seed muffin for breakfast may test positive for opioids, and if a person used cocaine 3 days ago, it is unlikely to show up in a urinalysis (UA) today. Hair samples can indicate that a person has been exposed to a substance, but not when, and can be affected by other environmental exposures. Record reviews, too, have limitations. They tell only the part of the story that is in official records, which can be inaccurate or incomplete.

Here are a few examples of instrument or data collection sections from journal articles.

Axis I substance use diagnoses (SUDs) were based on the results of the Structured Clinical Interview for DSM-III-R-Patient Edition with Psychotic Screen (SCID-P; Spitzer et al., 1990a). Axis II PD diagnoses were based on the results of the SCID-Personality Disorders (SCID-II; Spitzer et al., 1990b). The structured clinical interviews were administered by master's and doctoral-level interviewers, each of whom had received extensive training in the use of these instruments. The training included the viewing of SCID training videotapes, the observation of interviews being conducted by doctoral-level psychologists, and the administration of the instruments while being observed by a psychologist. (Thomas, Melchert, & Banker, 1999, pp. 271–272)

This article assumes that the reader has considerable knowledge about this instrument, because the authors provide virtually no description of it. Instead, they are referred to yet another journal article that describes the instrument. The reader would get the impression that the instrument must be fairly complex, since the training is extensive and the trainees are highly educated, but there is no information on the content of the items, how long it takes to administer, or whether the responses are open-ended or multiple choice. This article is found in the *Journal of Studies on Alcohol,* which is one of the scientifically rigorous research journals in the field and is primarily a vehicle for researchers to communicate with each other. It may be less likely to provide practical information for the substance abuse counselor than a more practice-oriented journal such as *Alcoholism Treatment Quarterly.* The next example gives a little more detail about the measures:

The study employed an interview schedule which had been piloted on over 100 injecting drug users and subsequently modified. Data on reliability and validity met established psychometric criteria. The interview schedule was developed specifically for the Australian drug use environment where different drugs are available to users (e.g., crack is as yet unavailable in Australia) and the legal and drug policy climate differs from other countries (e.g., possession of unused injection equipment is legal and free equipment is available from needle and syringe exchanges). Sections of the interview schedule covered demographics, drug use behavior, use of new equipment and reuse of old equipment, sharing of injection equipment, cleaning of injection equipment, disposal of used injection equipment, social context of injecting drug use, sexual history, knowledge and attitudes about HIV/AIDS, HIV/AIDS risk reduction behaviors, sources of HIV/AIDS information, HIV antibody testing, and modules on treatment and use of drugs in prison if appropriate. . . . Time intervals in the study were [the] last typical using month for drugs and for sexual behavior, past six months. (Dwyer et al., 1994, p. 381)

This article provides a much more detailed idea of what kind of information is collected and the social context of the study. There are no completely objective, trouble-free types of measurement in the field of substance abuse, so researchers determine which measures best fit the needs of the project and do not worry about perfection.

Research protocols or manuals are often used when researchers are studying treatment effectiveness. These are necessary in research, because every client must get the exact same treatment and the only way to do that is to have all people who are delivering the treatment follow exactly the same procedures. If the data collection includes an interview, then every question must be asked in exactly the same way for every client. If the intervention is to be delivered for 1 hour per day, then it must be given to every client for 1 hour each day. Any deviation from the protocol may bias the results. Many researchers prepare detailed manuals for carrying out the study, but no matter how comprehensive the instructions are, the people actually delivering the intervention may alter them in subtle or not so subtle ways. Counselors' attitudes about the intervention may get in the way in some cases. Maintaining the integrity of a treatment is called "fidelity."

For example, an agency is comparing a motivational interviewing to the standard approach ("treatment as usual," which often means that every counselor has his or her own way of doing things). Although the 12 counselors in the program are all given the same 3-hour training on this technique, they may use it in 12 different ways. One counselor will follow the manual to the letter, the next changes the wording of some of the intervention, and yet another uses the manual for 3 days and then decides to drop it. These events give researchers premature gray hair. Research protocols can be a bit like the childhood game of telephone. The protocol might become unrecognizable after it passes from one person to another, or from the manual to the group treatment room. If an agency commits to a research project, all the staff need to be committed to it, or only the committed ones should participate in delivering the experimental treatment. However, this latter scenario could introduce bias as well. If only the staff counselors who are committed to trying an experimental treatment deliver the treatment, and the ones who are not committed do their own thing, this may extend to factors beyond the research study. Maybe the more committed counselors are more open-minded and flexible than the noncommitted ones. Maybe they are more motivated and enthusiastic about their jobs, and the noncommitted ones are burned out. They may have different client outcomes regardless of the treatment. So if a study finds that motivational interviewing (MI) worked better than standard treatment, the reason might not be the MI technique, but better counselors. However, even the best counselors need periodic retraining on a protocol to maintain fidelity.

Conclusions

There are many factors that complicate studies of human behavior. Experimental research is one of the best ways to isolate one or a few variables to see what their effect is on the outcome, but it can be nearly impossible to control all the other factors that might influence the outcome. Working with human beings presents a challenge, because of the reliance on self-report data for many variables. There is no direct way to measure much of human motivation or psychological processing, and unfortunately, even the most educated and motivated research participant may provide inaccurate information for a variety of reasons—faulty memory, lack of insight into the problem, bias, being under the influence of a substance while being interviewed, being in withdrawal or not physically or cognitively well at the time of the study, and so on.

8

Data Analysis and Interpretation

Now for the part of the research process that many people fear or dread . . . the data analysis or statistical phase. Statistical analyses are a necessary component of most research. The statistical analysis reports the likelihood that a finding might be due to chance. It is not really important to know all the types of statistical analyses and how they work to understand the research process, but it is important to know why they are necessary and what the results mean. Statistical analyses come in two broad categories: descriptive and inferential. These two types of analyses will be described separately.

Descriptive Statistics

Descriptive statistics are widely used in everyday life, from advertising ("Get a 50% reduction in wrinkles with just 2 weeks of use"), public opinion polls ("80% of U.S. citizens favor comprehensive sex education"), the ballpark ("Cleveland's batting average as of July is .286."), and the doctor's office ("Your weight is at the 75th percentile"). Most people are familiar with descriptive statistics such as:

- the mean (the average of a set of scores),
- the median (the middle score in a range),
- the mode (the most frequently occurring score),

- the standard deviation (a measure of the average distance between scores, which shows if scores are grouped pretty close together or spread out over a large range),
- frequencies (how often each score appears), and
- correlations (the degree of relationship between two or more scores).

Some people believe that numbers do not lie and that descriptive statistics are completely objective. However, all statistics should be viewed with healthy skepticism, because they are only as good as the measures that they summarize, and they are prone to human judgment, manipulation, and interpretation. Used with caution, statistics have many important uses. The first application is with the properties of the instruments or measurements used in the study.

Reliability and Validity of Measurement Tools

Good research hinges on accurate measurement. To determine if the measures are statistically sound (also called psychometric properties), several different types of statistics are helpful. Reliability measures assess how consistent the measurement is. If client A gets a score of 100 today on an intelligence test, but a score of 75 tomorrow, there is a problem with the client or the intelligence test. Intelligence is supposed to be relatively stable and not fluctuate from day to day, so the measure might be unreliable. Validity refers to how well the assessment tool actually measures the concept of interest. If the intelligence tool is made up only of factual knowledge questions, one might question its validity.

Many types of reliability and validity are reported in the form of correlations. Correlations describe the degree of relatedness between two or more variables. A perfect positive correlation is +1.0. That means that as score number 1 goes up, score number 2 goes up in the same increments. If a researcher examines the number of drinks per week in relation to a measure of family dysfunction that ranges from 10, low dysfunction, to 40, very high dysfunction, as number of drinks goes up, so does the score on family dysfunction. Figure 8.1 shows the relationship in the form of a graph.

A perfect negative correlation would happen when as score 1 goes up, score 2 goes down (a correlation of −1.0). This time the variables are the number of drinks per week and emotional well-being. In this case, as the number of drinks goes up, the measure of well-being goes down (shown in Figure 8.2).

Perfect correlations never happen in the real world. Scores are correlated if there is some degree of tilt in the line drawn through the scores. Figure 8.3 shows scores that are not very correlated. There is a somewhat random

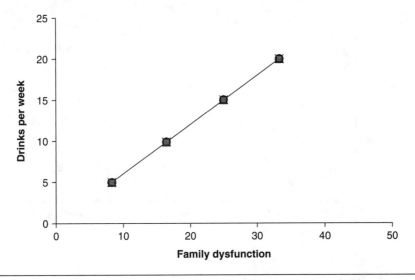

Figure 8.1   Relationship Between Number of Drinks per Week and Family Dysfunction

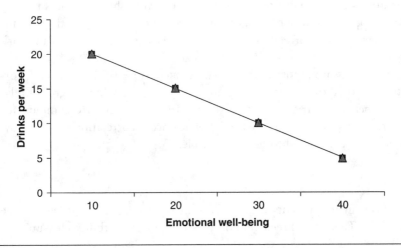

Figure 8.2   The Relationship Between Drinks per Week and Emotional Well-Being

pattern of scores in this distribution, and it would be impossible to draw a straight line through the scores.

There are a number of different types of correlations, including Pearson, Spearman, intraclass, and kappa coefficients, but the numbers that they yield

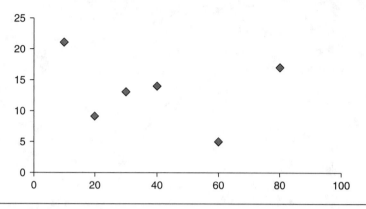

Figure 8.3   A Pattern of Weak or No Relationship Between Variables

are basically the same and they can be interpreted similarly. The interpretation of a correlation is similar whether the number refers to a reliability score, a validity measure, or the degree to which age is related to liver disease. Correlations do not indicate cause-and-effect relationships. There is no way of knowing which variable might cause the other, or if some third factor causes them both. Correlations indicate only how strongly related the variables are.

Correlations are reported as "r" scores, such as r = 0.71. In general, correlations of 0.90 to 1.0 are considered to indicate a very high degree of relationship between variables. Correlations of 0.70 to 0.89 are common for measures of psychological functioning, but once a correlation drops below that, it is not considered to be very reliable.

Reliability

Assessment instruments need to be somewhat consistent, at least in the short term. There are three commonly used types of reliability measures:

- Test-retest reliability
- Internal consistency (coefficient alpha and split-half reliability)
- Inter-rater reliability

For example, a researcher develops a new depression scale—it has 24 items that measure symptoms of depression such as apathy, crying, feeling worthless, and so on. She or he could test its reliability (how consistent it is) by comparing the first 12 items to the last 12 items, or the odd-numbered items to the even-numbered items (split-half reliability). No matter how the items are sliced up, about the same score (but not exactly the same score—that would be rare) would result. One minor problem with this approach is that there would probably be a slightly different correlation based on the first or second half or the odd/even split. A way to resolve this is to try all possible split halves (coefficient alpha) or compare people's scores at different points in time (test-retest).

Test-retest reliability can be collected in a short interval (the instrument given 2 days apart) or a longer interval, like 6 months. If the test measures a stable function, the scores should not be too different. However, if it measures something that often changes or sometimes changes, like feelings related to situational depression, the reliability scores will be lower. Some symptoms of depression during recovery are expected in many clients, but the symptoms generally will improve over time. Therefore, test-retest reliability data might be collected in a 1-week interval rather than a 3-month interval.

Inter-rater reliability is important for interviewer-administered instruments, structured interviews, or any measures based on clinical judgment. Good inter-rater reliability means that if one counselor gives the instrument to a client, there is a high likelihood that a different counselor giving the same instrument would get about the same score. Typically, an intraclass or kappa coefficient is used for inter-rater reliability to determine the interchangeability of the raters. (It does not matter which rater does the assessment because they are interchangeable.)

For all these types of reliability, the higher the correlation the better. A really good instrument has reliability measures of 0.90 or higher, but many psychological measurements are in the 0.80 range, because humans are not perfect or entirely consistent.

Validity

The second criterion of a good instrument is validity. How well does it measure the concept of interest to the study? If the depression scale contains items such as "Do you prefer chocolate ice cream to vanilla ice cream?" or "Do you consider yourself a good athlete?" it might not be as useful as a depression measure. There are several types of validity, including:

- **Content validity:** This is also known as face validity, which is present when experts examine the items to determine their relatedness to the overall concept. Experts on depression could be asked to review the new depression scale and give their opinion as to how well it measures the main components of depression.
- **Criterion validity:** The new depression measure could be compared to some gold standard, such as the *Diagnostic and Statistical Manual of*

Mental Disorders (DSM) criteria for depression. If both measures are given—the new depression scale and the DSM criteria—to a group of people and there is a correlation of .91 between the two scores, that means that people who got low scores on the new measure usually got low scores on the DSM criteria too. Now the researcher can be fairly certain that the new measure is valid because it appears to measure the same thing as the accepted measure.

• **Predictive validity:** The last type of validity is the hardest to do and is often ignored by researchers. Predictive validity is important, because if the instrument has no value in predicting some outcome, then why bother to use it? If the depression measure predicts the outcome of substance abuse treatment in some way, then it is useful to measure depression during treatment. If it has some influence on treatment outcome, then it has predictive validity. This, of course, requires a longitudinal study, which is why so many researchers fail to collect this information.

Some research is aimed solely at collecting reliability or validity data for some instrument. For example, Ross, Swinson, Doumani, and Larkin (1995) compared two different interviews for co-occurring disorders: the Computerized Diagnostic Interview Schedule (C-DIS) and the Structured Clinical Interview for the DSM (SCID). They divided 173 substance abusers in treatment into two groups assigned by a coin toss (random assignment) as follows:

Entry	1–2 weeks later with a different interviewer
Group 1: C-DIS then SCID	C-DIS
Group 2: SCID then C-DIS	SCID

The authors selected two groups because completing one interview about co-occurring disorders could affect the way the client responds to the second interview. Whenever two very similar measures are used, they should be counterbalanced. Here is part of the results section of that article:

> The C-DIS kappa values are generally in the good to excellent range (0.63 to 0.89) for the psychoactive substance use disorders but are lower for the other mental diagnoses. These kappas range from –0.05 (generalized anxiety) to 0.70 (simple phobia) . . . Generalized anxiety (–0.05), depressive disorder (0.12), and agoraphobia (0.20) all have unacceptably poor kappa coefficients. (Ross et al., 1995, pp. 175–176)

Kappa statistics are a type of correlation used to compare the agreement from one administration of a test to another. In this case, the C-DIS was taken by a client on a computer, and repeated 1 to 2 weeks later. Apparently the C-DIS relies too much on accuracy of memory for past events, since the clients often responded very differently the second time they took it. On the depression scale, there was only 12 percent agreement from time one to time two. This is important information for counselors to know—this instrument may not be very reliable, so why waste time giving it? Another possibility is that clients are not capable of providing very accurate information about their mental health in the first few days of entry into treatment. The instrument may have great psychometric characteristics, but if clients' trust levels, memory, attention, or other cognitive functions interfere with taking the test, the scores are probably not valid. In this case, there is no problem with the instrument, but rather with how it is used—it may not be appropriate to try to evaluate people when they are intoxicated, cognitively impaired, or psychiatrically unstable. Unfortunately, the research study cited above did not give any information on the cognitive or psychiatric status of the clients.

Many researchers do not report the reliability or validity of their instruments. If an instrument lacks reliability, change in scores from before an intervention to after the intervention is difficult to explain and could be due to random error. However, even a reliable instrument can be bad if it lacks validity. If a researcher decides to measure personality by making a plaster mold of people's heads and counting the number of bumps, he or she might be able to develop a very reliable system. But since there is no evidence that cranial bumps have anything to do with personality, the measure would be worthless. Most measures will not have such blatant flaws, but many of them have subtle problems. For example, many depression scales include items about physical complaints such as fatigue, body aches and pains, and difficulty sleeping. If the client or patient is an older adult with arthritis or a substance-dependent client undergoing withdrawal, these symptoms may not be related to depression at all. Think of the symptoms of withdrawal from different classes of drugs. Do they overlap with any other physical or mental health problems?

Interpreting Descriptive Statistics

The next section reviews the use of descriptive statistics. The first example comes from a study about child sexual abuse experiences and later substance abuse. The sample was drawn from randomly selected phone numbers in one state, and all the adult subjects were interviewed on the telephone. There were 50 men and 50 women. Table 8.1 shows some of the descriptive statistics by gender.

The numbers provide only some basic facts about men and women as a group—they do not explain the relationship between the numbers. For

Table 8.1   Fictitious Data on Child Abuse and Alcohol/Drug Problems

	Age (Mean and Range)	% Sexual Abuse	% Physical Abuse	% Lifetime Alcohol or Drug Problems
Men	33, 18–68	4%	15%	18%
Women	25, 18–49	22%	14%	12%

example, what percentage of the men who were sexually abused later developed alcohol or drug problems? Four percent of 50 is equal to two people. Since only two men were sexually abused in childhood, there are too few to study. Regarding the women, how can the researcher know what number of the 22 percent who experienced sexual abuse in childhood (which is only 11 women) also reported drug or alcohol problems in adulthood? What about the age difference between women and men? Is that significant?

There are other ways (cross-tabulations or frequency tables) of getting at these questions. Table 8.2 shows this kind of data for the women in the group.

Now this is a much more powerful descriptive finding. However, it still does not say that sexual abuse causes alcohol and drug problems, because four of the women who were sexually abused did not report any alcohol or drug problems (and this is not an experimental study). It does, however, show a potentially stronger relationship between the two variables and suggests that sexual abuse might be a risk factor for substance abuse. What might be mediating variables that led to substance abuse for some women but not for others?

Descriptive statistics can sometimes be misleading, especially when the data are "skewed" (lopsided) in some way. For example, recall the example of the human immunodeficiency virus (HIV) risk reduction intervention described earlier (Eldridge et al., 1997), where the authors noted that the "mean number of lifetime sex partners was 86.2 (SD = 181, median 27.5)" (p. 65). If the researchers reported only the mean, it would present a very

Table 8.2   Child Abuse and Alcohol/Drug Problems

Group	% With Alcohol or Drug Problems
Sexually abused (n = 11)	63%
Not sexually abused (n = 39)	7%

biased view of the sexual behavior of the group as a whole. The actual numbers are not available, but they might look something like Figure 8.4 (these are made-up data):

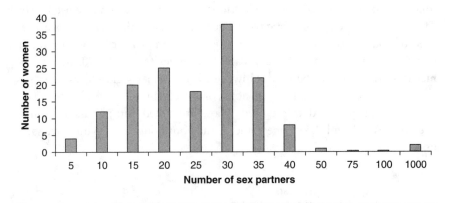

Figure 8.4   Frequency of Number of Lifetime Sex Partners in Substance-Abusing Women

The figure shows that just a few women threw off the whole distribution. It could be that two women, who were sex workers, each reported more than 1,000 sex partners. These two large numbers would pull the mean score to the right for the whole group. The authors realized that the distribution was skewed, so they reported the median score as well. This suggested that the majority of women had around 27 sex partners in their lifetimes (the median is the middle score in a distribution). Whenever the mean and median scores are this different (86 versus 27), and the standard deviation this large (181 was the average distance between scores, which were lifetime sex partners), the distribution must be skewed.

Inferential Statistics

The second class of statistical analyses is used to compare scores from two or more groups, compare a baseline score to a follow-up measure, and determine if the difference could be due to chance. For example, if African American clients score 63 on average on some measure, and European Americans score 60, is this a significant difference? If women participating in a self-esteem group score 50 before the group and 65 after the group, is that an indication of success of the treatment? Inferential statistics are only a tool for identifying whether a finding might be due to chance. Interpretation of the meaning of the result, or determining whether the difference is large enough to be considered important, is left to human judgment.

The inferential statistics are more complex than the descriptive stats. The following tables provide some definitions of the more commonly used tests. The type of inferential statistic performed depends on the types of measures used to characterize the variables. If they are numerical scales with a range of numbers, such as a loneliness scale that ranges from 0 to 50, then **parametric** statistics might be used. However, if the scales yield scores like "yes or no" or "alcohol dependent or not," or "age group 1, 2, or 3," then statistics for categorical data are used. These are called **non-parametric** statistics. Tables 8.3 and 8.4 define some of the commonly used parametric and non-parametric tests.

Table 8.3   Parametric Tests

t-test	Used to compare the means of two groups, or means before and after an intervention. For example, determining whether the severity of depression scores differs for men or women or if depression scores change from entry to exit from treatment. Reported as a "t" score.
ANOVA	Analysis of Variance (ANOVA) is used to compare the means of more than two groups. For example, are depression scores different for heterosexual men, heterosexual women, gay men, and lesbians? Reported as an "F" score.
Multiple Regression	Used to determine how much one measure or variable contributes to the score on another measure. Multiple regression analyses are a more complex variation of correlations and examine the relationships of more than two variables at once. For example, how much does age, IQ, or number of months sober contribute to or predict depression scores? There are several variations of regression, including stepwise, backward, and forward regression.
MANOVA	Multivariate Analysis of Variance (MANOVA) is used for the most complicated research designs that involve giving instruments over time, have complex groupings of subjects, or that control for the presence of one or more variables, such as age or IQ level.

Discriminant Analysis	This is a form of regression analysis used to make classification systems. For example, if we have some measure of drug and alcohol effects, we could use this to establish a cutoff score to classify people as addicted or not addicted.
Logistic Regression	Used when the outcome you wish to predict is dichotomous: "yes or no" or "abstinent or not abstinent." It is like multiple regression, except used to predict clients' probabilities of being in one group or another.
Survival Analysis	Survival analysis is like a multiple regression or a t-test but it is used when you want to analyze the time to some event, such as relapse. For example, you might be interested if criminal justice clients are more likely to relapse than clients from other referral sources. You might want to analyze whether or not the client relapses, i.e., is abstinent over a year follow-up. But some clients relapse early and some might not relapse until after the 1-year follow-up. So, you choose time-to-relapse as the dependent variable and do a survival analysis.
Analysis of Covariance	Most of the statistical procedures including ANOVA can include "covariates." These variables are used to control for noise, confounders, or other measured factors that might influence your results. For example, when comparing two treatment groups you might want to covary ("control for") the clients' age or duration of use. Some care should be used when including covariates in your analysis since they can strongly affect the interpretation. Also, they can give the appearance of making two groups the same on some confounding variable when they are not (fancy statistics cannot change apples to oranges).

Inferential statistics produce a p-value (probability value). These scores indicate whether the result, regardless of the type of inferential statistical procedure used, is statistically significant (less likely to be due to chance). Generally, a p-value of 0.05 or lower is considered to be evidence of a statistically significant result. This means that the probability of the finding being due to chance is only 5 in 100. If we are making a very important decision that could be costly if we are wrong, we might want to use a more stringent criterion, such as a p-value of 0.01 (1 in 100 chance of being wrong) or even 0.001 (1 in 1,000 chance of being wrong).

Table 8.4   Non-Parametric Tests

Chi-Square	Compares two frequencies. For example, if a depression measure is not a numerical scale, but depressed or not depressed, we could compare the percentage of women and men who were depressed. This is the non-parametric equivalent of a t-test and is the most widely used inferential statistic. Reported as a χ^2.
Goodness of Fit Testing	Used when there are more than two groups. It tests whether there are more or less in each category than expected. For example, if our agency served 89% white people, 5% African Americans, and 2% Latinos, is that different from the community figures? This is the non-parametric equivalent of an ANOVA and includes tests such as the Mann-Whitney U and the Wilcoxon Signed-Rank Test.
Mann-Whitney U and the Wilcoxon Rank-Sum Test	These are the non-parametric equivalent of a t-test and ANOVA and are useful when the data are skewed or otherwise not normal.

Other Statistical Methods

There are other statistical procedures that can be used to test theoretical models or look at the relationships among multiple variables. These include procedures such as **path analysis, factor analysis, odds ratios,** and **meta-analysis (effect size).**

Path analysis is sometimes used to determine how some event affects later events and to model and find mediators. Does peer pressure affect drinking directly, or does it change expectations that in turn affect actual drinking? This kind of analysis might help target where to focus prevention or treatment interventions.

Factor analysis is often used to determine if a measure is assessing only one concept or several. For example, that depression scale under development in the earlier section of this chapter might be a candidate for factor analysis. The researcher might find that there are two dimensions of depression that are assessed by that scale, one that is related to cognitions or feelings, and another that is related to physical symptoms.

Several procedures like logistic regression analyses produce **odds ratios** used to determine how much some factor increases the odds (i.e., chance) of some outcome. For example, if a woman does not drink any alcohol at all during pregnancy, her odds for having a child with some symptoms of fetal alcohol syndrome (FAS) would be very low. However, we might find that having two drinks per day increases the odds of these symptoms twofold (an odds ratio of 2.0) and that having five drinks per day increases the odds by 4.0 (four times higher than not drinking). There are a variety of similar types of statistics, for example, risk ratios and hazard ratios. Their interpretation is similar. A little care should be exercised when interpreting these kinds of ratios. When events have a low base rate, indicating that they are rare, the ratios can look impressively large, but a closer look at the actual percentages might reveal that the large-looking effect was caused by one or two people. If an agency has only one Native American client, an increase of just one more client doubles the rate of Native Americans represented in the agency. There is another consideration when interpreting p-values. If the authors tested a large number of variables, they may find a few "statistically significant" ones by chance. Consider throwing darts while you are blindfolded. The chance of accidentally getting a bull's-eye is slim. If you had enough darts, time, and patience, though, you might start getting a few.

Meta-analysis was developed to get an idea of how effective a treatment might be. Inferential statistics almost always present a p-value, but they do not indicate how successful a treatment was or how closely two things might be associated—they only tell the likelihood that the effects were driven by chance. Of course, it is important to know that the effect of some intervention was probably not a chance event, so the p-value is important. However, for policy and planning, it is necessary to know how well the treatment works. That is where "effect sizes" come in.

The problem presents, usually, with studies that are done on a large number of clients. Statistical analyses can become very sensitive and accurate with a big sample size. Thus, they might give small p-values for trivial or clinically unimportant effects. For example, suppose a state uses a particular curriculum for drivers arrested for a first offense of driving while intoxicated. A company offers them a new curriculum, saying that the new program "reduces second offenses by a statistically significant amount." The company did a study and even provided a p-value of 0.015 based on a total of 10,000 drivers (5,000 who received the old curriculum and 5,000 who received the new). Is the new curriculum better enough to warrant retooling the entire state's system of delivery? The answer is not evident from the existing data. If the original program resulted in 22 percent recidivism then, with that many drivers, a 2 percent reduction would produce a p-value of 0.015. That piece of information may provide more useful information—there appears to be a real reduction in recidivism, not due to chance, but it is not a large effect. The state may not want to make expensive changes in the system unless the drop in recidivism rates was larger.

There are many ways to present effect sizes. Which one is better depends on the situation. What is important to remember is

    a. p-values tell how "statistically significant" a result is but do not address how important an effect is; and

    b. Effect sizes help determine how "clinically significant" a result is.

Effect sizes are calculated by meta-analysis, which involves pooling several experimental studies on the same issue—for example, gathering all the experimental research available on the curriculum to address driving while intoxicated. This allows the researcher to average all the outcomes and determine if the overall effect is nonexistent, small, medium, or large.

Methods for Understanding Inferential Statistics

Researchers writing for each other often use considerable detail in the results sections of their articles, describing exactly how they analyzed the data. This is necessary if other researchers want to replicate the finding or be able to interpret the data. For most clinical purposes, however, the reader mainly wants to know what the researchers found, not how they went about finding it. An important piece of information to look for is the **p-values**. These numbers indicate that findings are not due to chance. As noted above, the p-value is often set at 0.05 for exploratory research, but might be set at 0.001 for important policy decisions. For example, if a county alcohol and drug program office wants to identify a list of evidence-based practices that they are confident produce significant improvements in outcomes, they might choose the stricter criterion. The stricter the criterion, however, the greater the chance of dismissing a result that is really valid and correct.

Example: Interpretation of a Clinical Trial

Bellack, Bennett, Gearon, Brown, and Yang (2006) developed a new intervention for clients with co-occurring severe and persistent mental illness (SPMI) and substance abuse. The article components are summarized as follows:

Sample

In the study, 293 clients were screened: of these, 175 met DSM-IV criteria for cocaine, heroin, or marijuana dependence, plus a SPMI. These 175 were characterized as follows: 66 percent were male, 75 percent were African

American, 38 percent were diagnosed with schizophrenia, 73 percent were cocaine dependent, and their mean age was 43 (standard deviation of 7.0).

Method

This was a clinical trial, so it met the core requirements of a clinical trial: subjects were randomly assigned to groups, there was an intervention, and there was a comparison group (treatment as usual). The two treatment conditions shared some characteristics: Both were administered in small groups twice a week for 6 months, and the trained therapists leading the groups followed treatment manuals. The two conditions were as follows:

1. Supportive Treatment for Addiction Recovery (STAR): This was the treatment as usual condition, and it consisted of group support with a little didactic education, but no formal curriculum and limited structure. UAs were obtained at each session, but no feedback was provided immediately about the UA.

2. Behavioral Treatment for Substance Abuse in SPMI (BTSAS): This was the experimental condition, developed specifically for this study using a harm reduction theoretical model. In addition to the twice-weekly group sessions, there were three individual motivational interviewing (MI) sessions to increase motivation; incentives for clean UAs ($1.50 to $3.50 per session, increasing by 50-cent increments for successive clean UAs, and resetting back to $1.50 after a dirty UA), UA results were announced in group to elicit positive support for clean UAs, and clients were taught coping skills, relapse prevention, and social skills training.

Outcome Measures

There were two major outcome measures:

1. UAs at each treatment session

2. Treatment dropout rates (dropout was defined as missing eight consecutive sessions)

Secondary outcome measures included 4- and 8-week abstinence rates; the number of treatment sessions attended; and a variety of self-report measures, including the Addiction Severity Index (ASI), a quality-of-life scale, and a substance use survey for schizophrenia.

Results

One concern in interpreting the results of any study is the attrition rate. The authors reported that of the 175 enrolled, 129 individuals attended at least one session, and 110 became engaged in treatment: 35 percent of those in treatment as usual and 57 percent of those in BTSAS completed the treatment. Is that an acceptable attrition rate? Table 8.5 shows two of the results, indicating that the BTSAS intervention produced significantly better outcomes than treatment as usual. Is the difference of practical significance as well if 59 percent of BTSAS clients had clean UAs at the end of treatment compared to 25 percent of clients in treatment as usual? Probably, yes, the rate of abstinence is more than double. The proportion data could be analyzed via an ANOVA, resulting in an F score, whereas the 4-week block of clean UAs was a yes or no response, thus analyzed via a chi square. However, both results provide a p-value, allowing consideration of the likelihood that the result is due to chance. In both cases, the chance is less than 1 in 1,000. The authors noted, "We examined 4-week and 8-week periods during which subjects attended every session, and these data show a pronounced advantage for BTSAS. Significantly more subjects in BTSAS had at least one 4-week block of continuous abstinence (54.1% vs. 16.3%, $\chi^2 = 15.3$, p < .001)" (Bellack et al., 2006, p. 430). The BTSAS subjects did better on nearly every outcome measured. The authors also reported the cost of the UA contingency management—it cost about $60 per subject on average, with a range of 0 to $168.50. The total cost of the program per person was $372, and the authors reported that "the benefits include a 23% reduction in outpatient admissions" (p. 431).

Interpretation/Application

While the study has fairly clear-cut, significant differences between the BTSAS and treatment as usual on all the outcome measures, would an agency adopt this intervention based on this study? Some of the limitations

Table 8.5   Results From Bellack et al. (2006)

Outcome	BTSAS (n = 61)	STAR (n = 49)	Statistic	p-value
Proportion of clean UAs	0.589	0.247	F = 16.05	<.001
Having at least one 4-week block of clean UAs	54%	16%	$\chi^2 = 15.3$	<.001

are: the authors developed the intervention and thus are not impartial; a small sample in only one geographic region; fairly large attrition; and no follow-up data reported. The only circumstance in which one might consider adopting this intervention based only on one small study is if the agency had a dire need for an intervention, had a similar client base to the participants in the study, and considered it an experimental situation and gathered some kind of outcome data about it.

In general, the best strategy for getting all the information you need from a research article is to read the abstract carefully—it summarizes the study. Then read the introduction and skim the literature review for the background information, determine if the sample is comparable to the agency's clients (to know if the findings might generalize to your work situation), skim the results, and read the discussion section carefully. The discussion section almost always includes some statements about the implications of the study for the field.

The results present the particular findings of the study, and the discussion talks about generalities. Read carefully to make sure that the results correspond to the discussion. For example, in the discussion the authors might conclude that their new treatment is successful. However, the results section reports that the treatment reduced the amount that clients drank but also reduced the number of clients who were abstinent. Was the treatment successful? It seems to depend on the particular definition. Some researchers go beyond their data in the discussion section.

Conclusions

Data analysis can be complicated in terms of procedure, but not so complicated in terms of interpretation. Once readers become accustomed to looking for p-values and/or effect sizes, the results sections of articles become less overwhelming. Data analysis is simply a tool, however, and it is still up to human judgment to interpret what the findings mean.

9

Qualitative Research, Dissemination, and Funding

This final chapter on research processes deals with qualitative research methods, dissemination of research findings, and funding sources for research.

Introduction to Qualitative Research

The previous chapters focused on quantitative analyses—based on numbers, ratings, or rankings of some kind. Qualitative methods are more subjective (although remember that interpreting numbers is not entirely objective either), such as trying to understand people's feelings or the meanings that they attach to their experiences. There is no attempt to identify "the truth," but rather to understand something about individuals' perceptions, experiences, or reactions to specific events. Qualitative research is valuable when we need to know opinions that might affect treatment (clients' perceptions of barriers to treatment, for example) or when little is known about some issue, such as, "What does drug craving really feel like?" Qualitative research is not of help in identifying which treatment interventions work best, but may be helpful in identifying the reasons *why* the treatment works or does not work.

Research studies often use a combination of quantitative and qualitative methods for a more thorough understanding of the issues. Qualitative research used to be considered "soft science" and quantitative research "hard science," but in reality quantitative research, with its focus on numbers and classification, cannot answer all the questions that need to be addressed in order to improve substance abuse treatment services. Much of human experience is subjective and qualitative in nature. Qualitative data make the subject come to life and adds richness and texture to the research literature.

Qualitative Methods

Qualitative research is not as driven by hypotheses or research questions as is quantitative research, so the research question might be very open-ended, such as, "What draws adolescents to smoking?" or "How do cocaine-dependent women view their relationships with their children?" There are variables, but there is no manipulation of any variables, so no real independent variable per se, and often there is no control or comparison group. Sometimes the purpose of the research is to further refine definitions for variables, such as drug craving or parenting from prison, or treatment motivation—what do these things mean to individuals who experience them? Are there common themes in the experience?

Samples are often smaller in qualitative studies, because the goal is for depth of information rather than gathering a little info from a lot of people. Therefore, random population studies or even concerns about representativeness are less important. Instead, samples are chosen for particular qualities—respondents who can provide information on the topic of interest, such as mothers of adolescent cocaine users, or men whose fathers were alcoholics. The small number of participants are given more intensive interviews and data collection.

The procedures are generally face-to-face or phone interviews and/or naturalistic observations in the field. Sometimes the interviews are quite structured (the researcher asks all the participants the same questions in exactly the same way), but sometimes they are much more open-ended and loose, allowing participants to tell their stories in their own words and in their own rhythms. Because qualitative research is more deliberately subjective, attention is paid to the context and the particular interactions of the researcher, the participant, and the audience for the work. If the researcher is conducting interviews or is a participant-observer in a setting, the researcher him- or herself is an instrument of the study. Questions such as "How will participants respond to me as the researcher or interviewer?" are important considerations. In this way, qualitative researchers are a lot like clinicians, who must worry about building rapport with participants or clients in order to get full and truthful answers from them while honoring their privacy and protecting their confidentiality.

The product of the research, or the "data," is generally words to describe participants' experiences or their actions, so statistics are not so important in the analysis. Descriptive statistics may be used to inform readers about the characteristics of the people studied, but no inferential statistics are used. Instead, the most common procedure for analysis is called content analysis. This involves gathering transcripts of all the interviews and searching for common themes. For example, Hall (1996) described a qualitative method called narrative analysis:

> Narrative is naturalistic, a form of everyday communication. In naturalistic studies of human conditions, in-depth experiential data from selected individuals is more valued than is a large sample (Morse, 1989). Through community-based purposive sampling in San Francisco, California, during 1990 and 1991, 35 lesbians recovering from alcohol problems participated in this study. . . . The researcher conducted and audiotaped a two hour, semi-structured interview with each participant, usually in the participant's home. . . . Interview topics were: defining alcohol use as a problem, seeking help, barriers to recovery, interacting with health care providers, participating in Alcoholics Anonymous (AA) and maintaining recovery. Open-ended questions were used and interruption of participants was purposefully avoided. . . . This enhanced mutuality, rapport, and subjective validity of participants' conversations. . . . Verbatim transcripts were used in the analysis. (Hall, 1996, pp. 230–231)

The transcripts were then reviewed, and consistent themes were identified. The results section of a qualitative article will often provide verbatim quotations from participants to allow the reader to compare the themes. For example, Hall puts the participants' words in quotation marks when she describes some of these themes:

> Alcohol and drugs were described as helpful in facilitating social and sexual interactions with other women during the lesbian "coming out" phase for both abused and nonabused groups. In the CSA (childhood sexual abuse) subsample, however, alcohol was also used to "numb feelings" or "not remember" past trauma. . . . The CSA survivors said they used alcohol to "function" in their daily lives, drinking constantly to feel "normal." (Hall, 1996, p. 233)

Even though the sample sizes are usually pretty small, qualitative data give us more of a flavor of what it feels like to be alcohol-dependent or to be a survivor of sexual abuse. Many research studies use a combination of quantitative and qualitative data collection methods. Often people's perceptions of events are more important than reality; therefore, these subjective studies can offer insight into clients' thinking processes and help identify irrational patterns of thinking, styles of coping, or common experiences. The qualitative interviews or questions may provide insight into the respondents' answers on the quantitative measures. The richness of a client's own words can convey an idea in a much more powerful way than a chart or graph. For example, one participant in a research study on women drug users said:

> The funny thing is that after about two weeks to three weeks you think you are cured. "I mean you are like, "I'm never going to use again, I'm cured." But you're not. Do you know what I mean? That's just the start of your recovery. After three weeks when your head starts thinking a bit straighter, that is just really the start of the hard times to come. The first three weeks are nothing compared to what is to come if you follow through because there's all the uncertainties. And everyone thinks 'cause you are over withdrawals and you don't need a hit that you should be all right. But I don't think so many people understand that that's when it really starts getting frightening. (Taylor, 1993, pp. 144–145)

This statement gives some very practical ideas to substance abuse counselors—that 2 to 3 weeks after withdrawal can be a crucial relapse time. This concept may have been hard to capture in a quantitative questionnaire.

Another Example of Qualitative Research in Substance Abuse

Jessup, Humphreys, Brindis, and Lee (2003) wanted to understand the impact of public policies that attempt to stop or reduce maternal drug use. They recruited 36 women from 15 residential treatment programs for pregnant and parenting women in northern California: 12 who were pregnant and 24 who had had a child in the past year. The descriptive statistics used to give information about the 36 women indicated that their mean gestational age at entry to substance abuse treatment was 17 weeks (with a standard deviation of 14.4 weeks); that 35 of the 36 women (97 percent) had sought some type of prenatal care; and that 19 (53 percent) had one or more obstetric and/or medical complication related to drug use during their pregnancies. The women had a mean of 18 weeks of clean and sober time at the time of the interview (standard deviation of 20). The analysis of the interview data resulted in verbatim quotations that illustrated the main themes, such as:

> Knowing that they were gonna test me for drugs, that's what scared me . . . that's why I didn't go to prenatal care . . . I didn't want to lose my baby (Emily, a 23 year old heroin user). (Jessup et al., 2003, p. 291)

. . . they told me if I come three times dirty that . . . when I had my baby, they was gonna take my baby (Ivy, 22 year old mother of two). (Jessup et al., 2003, p. 292)

This is a common way to present qualitative data—verbatim quotations with a little demographic information about the interviewee to provide more context. The authors made this conclusion:

Findings from this study support other research on fear as an extrinsic barrier for pregnant drug dependent women, hastening the "flight from care." . . . Participant's adaptive strategies in response to fear suggest that the desire for child custody and concern for fetal and child well-being was a priority that motivated care seeking despite extrinsic barriers perceived to be threatening to their safety and autonomy. (Jessup et al., 2003, p. 296)

Qualitative findings may be used to generate hypotheses, develop an intervention, develop a quantitative instrument, or evaluate a program or intervention.

Data Reporting and Dissemination

The review of research has focused on research reported in the form of journal articles, because publication in peer-reviewed journals is the primary way that academic institutions evaluate the work of researchers. Figure 9.1 shows some of the research-oriented journals in the field. These are the journals that specialize in substance abuse topics. However, researchers may publish their findings about substance abuse in general medical, psychiatric, public health, psychological, or other social science journals as well, as a quick glance through the References for this book will indicate.

"Publish or perish" for academics means peer-reviewed journals, not newsletters, lay press articles, or even chapters in books. This sad reality means that most researchers write primarily for other researchers and rarely translate their research into a form that might be more directly useful to the substance abuse provider. However, there are other sources of information that do some of that synthesis work. Reviews of the literature in journals, books, and chapters in books often summarize the research in some area, so that readers do not have to read dozens of research articles. The federal government issues a number of publications that are based on research but aimed at the provider audience, such as the Center for Substance Abuse Treatment's TIPs (Treatment Improvement Protocols) and TAPs (Technical

---

Addiction
Addiction Research
Addiction Research and Theory
Addictive Behaviors
Alcohol
Alcohol Health and Research World *
Alcoholism: Clinical and Experimental Research
Alcoholism Treatment Quarterly *
American Journal of Drug and Alcohol Abuse
British Journal of Addiction
Contemporary Drug Problems
Drug and Alcohol Dependence
Journal of Addictions Nursing
Journal of Addictive Diseases
Journal of Drug Issues
Journal of Psychoactive Drugs
Journal of Studies on Alcohol
Journal of Substance Abuse
Journal of Substance Abuse Treatment
Psychology of Addictive Behaviors
Nicotine and Tobacco Research
Substance Abuse
Substance Abuse Treatment, Prevention, and Policy
Substance Use and Misuse
Tobacco Control

Figure 9.1   Selected Substance Abuse Research Journals

* More oriented to practitioners

Assistance Publications) series. Figure 9.2 lists some of the recent TIPs titles. Many providers have some of these on their shelves—they focus on different topics or various client populations and translate the research on the topic. Some of these sources are peer-reviewed and some are not. TIPs and TAPs are developed via consensus panels of researchers, providers, and policy-makers who are knowledgeable about the topic. In this sense, most of the TIPs and TAPs series are more like clinical practice guidelines than they are like evidence-based practices.

Web sites are another source of information, but the Internet is not well regulated, and it sometimes becomes difficult to sift the accurate information from someone's personal opinions. It is best to stay with federal or private foundations that focus on substance abuse. The Resources section at the end of the References for this book lists some of these Web sites. In general, Web sites that end with .edu (education sites) or .gov (government sites) are the

- **TIP 45:** Detoxification and Substance Abuse Treatment

  https://ncadistore.samhsa.gov/catalog/productDetails.aspx?ProductID=17398

  This TIP provides clinicians with the latest information on detoxification: the physiology of withdrawal, pharmacologic advances in the management of withdrawal, patient placement procedures, and managing detoxification services within comprehensive systems of care. The publication emphasizes that by itself, detoxification does not constitute complete substance abuse treatment, and it identifies the necessity for linking patients in detoxification with substance abuse treatment services. TIP 45 is a revision of TIP 19, Detoxification From Alcohol and Other Drugs.

- **TIP 44:** Substance Abuse Treatment for Adults in the Criminal Justice System

  http://www.ncbi.nlm.nih.gov/books/bv.fcgi?rid=hstat5.chapter.80017

  This TIP presents clinical guidelines to help substance abuse treatment counselors address issues that arise from their clients' status in the criminal justice system. In addition, it will aid personnel in the criminal justice system in understanding and addressing the challenges of working with offenders with substance use disorders. This new TIP replaces three TIPs: TIP 7, Screening and Assessment for Alcohol and Other Drug Abuse Among Adults in the Criminal Justice System; TIP 12, Combining Substance Abuse Treatment With Intermediate Sanctions for Adults in the Criminal Justice System; and TIP 17, Planning for Alcohol and Other Drug Abuse Treatment for Adults in the Criminal Justice System.

- **TIP 43:** Medication-Assisted Treatment for Opioid Addiction in Opioid Treatment Programs

  http://www.ncbi.nlm.nih.gov/books/bv.fcgi?rid=hstat5.chapter.82676

  TIP 43 provides treatment providers, physicians, and other medical personnel with the latest information on medication-assisted treatment for people addicted to opiates, largely prescription narcotics or heroin. The TIP emphasizes the importance of supportive services such as counseling, mental health, and other medical services, and vocational rehabilitation in facilitating recovery for patients receiving mediation-assisted treatment. The document outlines best practices in the use of methadone, buprenorphine, and naltrexone, including appropriate doses of medication, medically supervised withdrawal, medication maintenance, tapering off of treatment medications, associated medical problems, treatment for multiple substance use, and other crucial aspects of treatment for those who are addicted to opiates.

- **TIP 42:** Substance Abuse Treatment for Persons With Co-Occurring Disorders

  http://www.ncbi.nlm.nih.gov/books/bv.fcgi?rid=hstat5.chapter.74073

  TIP 42 provides information about new developments in the rapidly growing field of co-occurring substance use and mental disorders and captures the state of the art in the treatment of people with co-occurring disorders. The TIP contains chapters on terminology, assessment, treatment strategies, and

(Continued)

Figure 9.2   Recent CSAT Treatment Improvement Protocols

models, and an overview of specific mental disorders and cross-cutting issues, such as suicidality and nicotine dependence. The TIP's appendices provide additional information on topics such as specific mental disorders, emerging models of treatment, common medications, screening and assessment instruments, dual recovery mutual self-help programs, and other resources for consumers and providers, as well as confidentiality issues.

- **TIP 41:** Substance Abuse Treatment: Group Therapy

  http://www.ncbi.nlm.nih.gov/books/bv.fcgi?rid=hstat5.chapter.78366

  This TIP contains detailed information about group therapy modalities, techniques, and practices that are valuable to substance abuse treatment counselors as well as supervisors and trainers of counselors. It describes five group models that are common in substance abuse treatment.

- **TIP 40:** Clinical Guidelines for the Use of Buprenorphine in the Treatment of Opioid Addiction

  http://www.ncbi.nlm.nih.gov/books/bv.fcgi?rid=hstat5.chapter.72248

  This TIP provides consensus- and evidence-based guidance on the use of buprenorphine, a new option for the treatment of opioid addiction. The goal of this TIP is to provide information that physicians can use to make practical and informed decisions about the use of buprenorphine to treat opioid addiction. The guidelines address a number of topic areas related to this goal, including the physiology and pharmacology of opioids, opioid addiction, and treatment with buprenorphine; the screening and assessment of opioid addiction problems; detailed protocols for opioid addiction treatment with buprenorphine; management of special populations; and policies and procedures related to office-based opioid addiction treatment under the paradigm established by the Drug Addiction Treatment Act of 2000. This TIP represents another step by CSAT toward its goal of bringing national leaders together to improve substance use disorder treatment in the United States.

- **TIP 39:** Substance Abuse Treatment and Family Therapy

  http://www.ncbi.nlm.nih.gov/books/bv.fcgi?rid=hstat5.chapter.70382

  This TIP addresses how substance abuse affects the entire family and how substance abuse treatment providers can use principles from family therapy to change the interactions among family members. The TIP provides basic information about family therapy for substance abuse treatment professionals and basic information about substance abuse treatment for family therapists. The TIP presents the models, techniques, and principles of family therapy, with special attention to the stages of motivation as well as to treatment and recovery. Discussion also focuses on clinical decision making and training, supervision, cultural considerations, specific populations, funding, and research. The TIP further identifies future directions for both research and clinical practice.

Figure 9.2 (Continued)

- **TIP 38:** Integrating Substance Abuse Treatment and Vocational Services

  http://www.ncbi.nlm.nih.gov/books/bv.fcgi?rid=hstat5.chapter.68228

  Employment has been positively correlated with retention in treatment. By holding a job, a client establishes a legal source of income, structured use of time, and improved self-esteem, which in turn may reduce substance use and criminal activity. Unemployment and substance abuse may be intertwined long before an individual seeks treatment. Although the average educational level of individuals with substance abuse disorders is comparable to that of the general U.S. population, people who use substances are far more likely to be unemployed or underemployed than people who do not use substances. According to the U.S. Census Bureau, employment rates for the non-substance-using population ranged from 72.3 percent in 1980 to 76.8 percent in 1991. However, employment rates of the population with substance abuse problems before admission or at admission to treatment have remained at relatively stable, low levels since 1970, ranging from 15 to 30 percent. Most of the research on the employment rates of persons with substance abuse disorders has focused on opiate- (usually heroin-) dependent persons, and employment rates for other substance users may vary. The data clearly indicate the need for interventions to improve employment rates among this population in treatment and recovery.

- **TIP 37:** Substance Abuse Treatment for Persons With HIV/AIDS

  http://www.ncbi.nlm.nih.gov/books/bv.fcgi?rid=hstat5.chapter.64746

  While AIDS remains a deadly disease, since TIP 15 was published in 1995 new treatment approaches have extended the length and quality of survival for those with HIV. This longer-term survival requires innovative substance abuse treatment that encourages people with HIV/AIDS to seek substance abuse treatment and maintain recovery. TIP 37 provides a comprehensive overview of how the HIV/AIDS epidemic requires substance abuse treatment professionals to attend to the multiple needs of their clients with HIV/AIDS: substance abuse and other medical, behavioral, psychological, and social needs. TIP 37 reviews the history, transmission, and progression of HIV/AIDS and describes the changes in epidemiology since 1995. It reports on the current state of medical and mental health treatment and how this affects people with substance abuse disorders and HIV/AIDS. Counseling issues are addressed, including staff attitudes, screening, and issues specific to the client with substance abuse disorders and HIV/AIDS. The TIP also examines ethical and legal issues of particular import to both substance abuse treatment providers and their clients with HIV/AIDS, and concludes with an overview of funding sources and grant-writing guidelines.

- **TIP 36:** Substance Abuse Treatment Responding to Child Abuse and Neglect Issues

  http://www.ncbi.nlm.nih.gov/books/bv.fcgi?rid=hstat5.chapter.63145

  The effects of childhood abuse and neglect perpetrated by family members and the intergenerational transmission of the cycle of substance abuse and

(Continued)

child abuse and neglect are the focus of this TIP. The seven chapters discuss working with child abuse and neglect issues; screening and assessing adults for childhood abuse and neglect; comprehensive treatment for adult survivors; therapeutic issues for counselors; the substance-dependent client as parent/caregiver; legal responsibilities; and emerging and continuing issues. The closing recommendations include screening assessment protocol and issues for counselors.

- **TIP 35:** Enhancing Motivation for Change in Substance Abuse Treatment

  http://www.ncbi.nlm.nih.gov/books/bv.fcgi?rid=hstat5.chapter.61302

  This TIP shows how substance abuse treatment staff can influence change by developing a therapeutic relationship that respects and builds on the client's autonomy and, at the same time, makes the treatment clinician a partner in the change process.

- **TIP 34:** Brief Interventions and Brief Therapies for Substance Abuse Treatment

  http://www.ncbi.nlm.nih.gov/books/bv.fcgi?rid=hstat5.chapter.59192

  An increasing number of individuals are presenting with substance abuse disorders while at the same time, recent changes in the health care delivery system are placing funding and time constraints on clinicians. The need for cost-effective services to address substance use disorders is great. As a result, clinicians, researchers, and policymakers are turning their attention toward brief interventions and therapies. An increasing body of literature confirms the effectiveness of brief approaches in substance abuse treatment. This TIP links research to practice by providing clinicians with information on these innovative and shorter forms of treatment for selected populations of substance-using individuals.

- **TIP 33:** Treatment for Stimulant Use Disorders

  http://www.ncbi.nlm.nih.gov/books/bv.fcgi?rid=hstat5.chapter.57310

  Over the past 20 years, stimulant use in the United States has risen dramatically. Consequently, clinicians, treatment program administrators, and criminal justice system officials must be prepared to address problems and needs specific to this population. This TIP presents information on the nature and extent of cocaine and methamphetamine abuse, and translates findings from clinical studies into practical treatment guidelines.

Figure 9.2 (Continued)

most likely to contain accurate information. Commercial sites (.com) are generally trying to sell products, so the buyer must beware. Sites sponsored by organizations (.org) are a mixed bag—some are legitimate sites with very accurate and up-to-date information, and others are airing opinions disguised as fact.

Beware also of information obtained from "sound bites" in newspapers, magazines, or TV news programs. These often simplify the research into one or two interesting sentences and completely ignore the methodological issues or sample questions. For example, the media blitz announcing that moderate alcohol intake is good for the heart is a much too simplified version of the reality. While this may be true for a small subset of society, there are other groups for whom any alcohol intake increases other health risks to the point that they may cancel out any benefits to the heart (for example, women of all ages, and adults over the age of 65).

Funding Sources

There are many different forms of funding sources in substance abuse research. Some of the block grant money given by the federal government is reserved for research or evaluation projects. This money comes from the Substance Abuse and Mental Health Services Administration (SAMHSA) agencies such as the Center for Substance Abuse Treatment and the Center for Substance Abuse Prevention. These agencies are primarily concerned with practical, applied research in local communities. In the past, SAMHSA funded some applied research studies, but recently, changes in procedures have eliminated much of their discretion to fund such programs and have limited their scope to evaluation projects. Other federal agencies, such as the National Institute on Drug Abuse (NIDA) and the National Institute on Alcohol Abuse and Alcoholism (NIAAA) generally fund basic research projects with rigorous experimental designs. These National Institutes of Health (NIH) agencies were historically less interested in application of their findings to the field, although this is beginning to change as the public demands to know what is done with the billions of dollars spent on basic research. The political issues that created two separate agencies—one focused on alcohol and the other on illicit drugs—contribute to an artificial division in the field. Some researchers also receive funding for substance abuse–related research through other federal agencies, such as the Centers for Disease Control and Prevention (CDC), the Center for Nursing Research, or the National Institute of Mental Health (NIMH). The National Institute of Justice also funds substance abuse research.

Pharmaceutical companies may fund research on drug treatments for substance abuse. There are many ethical considerations involved in the decision about whether to accept money from a company that is invested in getting positive results. Also, there is little incentive for drug companies to fund studies of behavioral treatments, even when comparing a pharmacological treatment to a behavioral treatment. It is in their best interest to show that drugs work better than behavioral treatments.

There are also private foundations that fund research projects. For example, the Robert Wood Johnson Foundation funds studies that examine substance abuse policies, as well as the Paths to Recovery program that focuses on practice improvements in the substance abuse treatment field. The American Legacy Foundation was created from tobacco settlement money and funds demonstration projects and applied research related to tobacco. There are also state and local sources of funding. It can be difficult to identify all the possible sources of funding for research. However, universities usually have offices of research devoted to keeping researchers up to date on funding opportunities. The Foundation Center is also a good resource for identifying research opportunities (http://foundationcenter.org/). A healthy collaboration between providers and researchers would link the researchers with the funding sources and grant-writing skills to the providers with the practical knowledge and access to research participants.

Conclusions

Qualitative research designs are a vital component of an evidence-based practice movement, and are particularly useful at the beginning, in theory and intervention development, and again later in the evaluation of the intervention, identifying what works about the intervention, and how to implement it. Qualitative research adds the human voice to research.

The sections on research dissemination and funding highlight some of the challenges to the field. The major sources of research dissemination are not user-friendly to the clinician. Other ways of rapid dissemination or synthesizing of large bodies of research are needed. Clinical guidelines, such as TIPs, are useful but may take years to produce. Creative use of Web sites that can be updated regularly might be more helpful.

Finally, funding sources for substance abuse treatment research are somewhat limited. Historically, the division of NIDA and NIAAA is contrary to the polydrug nature of the field and can create artificial distinctions where none truly exists. The reduction in funding available through SAMHSA for applied research has stifled the study of implementation of evidence-based practices. The schisms between basic and applied research; efficacy and effectiveness; and knowledge development and implementation need to be breached.

10

Conclusions and Future Directions

The complex and changing demands of practice will almost always outstrip the scientific knowledge base and treatment guidelines, no matter how well developed or scientifically sound, will never totally eliminate the need for experienced clinical judgment. But that reality should not deter the use of science to inform and guide practice to the extent possible. (Tucker & Roth, 2006, p. 920)

As substance abuse treatment efficacy and effectiveness research increases in both the number of studies and in their scientific rigor, we can begin to identify practices that work—or do not work—with particular subgroups of clients, paying attention to human diversity. However, the identification of effective practices is only one small step in improving substance abuse treatment delivery. At this juncture, it is critical to study the processes by which these new practices can become incorporated into the field, and how alterations or modifications of these practices affect outcomes. There is a great need in the field for studies of the implementation or adoption phase of research-based practices. This type of research is as important as research that identifies practices that work in ideal settings. In addition, the emphasis on the science base and implementing research into practice must be balanced with issues related to counselor competencies and training, and client and community needs and values.

Barriers to Conducting Research in Substance Abuse Treatment and Prevention Agencies

It has become quite clear that it is difficult to do controlled research in community-based treatment programs, but crucial that the barriers to such research be reduced. The study of implementation of evidence-based practice hinges on testing sites in the real world, and any type of research emanating from practice settings will have some of the best practical application to the field. There are barriers from both the researcher and provider perspectives that need to be addressed.

Researchers often feel that substance abuse counselors have negative attitudes about research, or lack basic knowledge of the research process, making the counselors less willing or able to participate in research. Sometimes researchers think that counselors resist change or think that the research threatens their jobs. (The research might reveal that their current practices are ineffective, for example.) Researchers mourn the loss of control that they experience when they do research in a practice setting. In a laboratory or university setting, they hire and train all the research staff and closely supervise them throughout the process. In a lab or university setting, space, degree of privacy, and many other factors can be controlled. This is harder to do in a clinical setting. Researchers need to learn better ways to work with providers and view them as part of the research team rather than as potential obstacles to conducting research.

From the viewpoint of a provider, researchers often do not understand the demands of the provider organization, the lack of time to add additional assessments or treatments, or how short-staffed and short on space most agencies are. The turnover of staff in substance abuse counseling is very high, with frequent demands on old staff to train and supervise new members. This leaves little time for research. Some researchers may also have unrealistic expectations about client characteristics or participation in research. For example, one researcher may wish to study the effects of cocaine on pregnancy. The staff members are directed to screen all incoming clients and assign those who use only cocaine and no other substances to a special treatment group. This researcher is clearly out of touch with reality and would end up with very few subjects. Substance abuse counselors are in the best position to identify the research priorities in the field and to help researchers develop studies that are realistic and feasible.

The obvious solution to this problem is to have researchers and providers work together from the beginning—in the identification of relevant research questions, designing and carrying out the study, and finally, disseminating the results. This will result in research questions that are more relevant to the participating agency and ultimately, the field; a research design that is realistic, implementable, and more likely to succeed; and better dissemination of the findings. The researcher can write the inevitable research jargon-laden report for a peer-reviewed journal, but can also work with providers to do presentations for the agency or at provider conferences about their findings. Substance abuse providers who have been involved in the research from the beginning will be better able to understand how to implement the findings. Recommendations for fostering research-practice collaborations are offered later in this chapter.

Major Themes Identified in This Book

The review of the state of the art of the evidence-based practice movement can be summarized through a few general themes, or conclusions about where the field stands at this point in time. These themes are detailed below, followed by some recommendations for moving the field ahead in a strategic, well-planned way.

Treatment effectiveness research in the substance abuse field is still in its infancy.

Even though there are randomized clinical trials of some treatment practices (mostly efficacy trials), only a handful of treatment approaches have been subjected to the rigorous test of a clinical trial. The National Institute on Drug Abuse (NIDA) Clinical Trials Network is one positive step in the direction of increasing the number of approaches subjected to clinical trials. However, the field may be several years from being able to say with confidence that any treatment method is superior to another. In addition, too much reliance on clinical trial data may limit the scope of practice and stifle the development of innovative new practices. At this point, a broader definition of research evidence than just clinical trials may be needed.

There is no one evidence-based practice that is clearly superior to others.

There are a variety of pharmacological and behavioral therapies with essentially equivalent effects on outcomes. However, there is less information on cost-effectiveness and practicality issues that might make some practices more likely to be implemented in community-based treatment agencies. There is no doubt that treatment works, but it is unlikely that the field will ever be able to identify a few practices that work best in all settings with all types of clients. There will always be room for a variety of different theoretical approaches that match counselor styles and client preferences. Ultimately, treatment agencies will have a menu of practices that are effective for different subpopulations or with different presenting problems.

Effective practices are not well implemented in the field.

The effective practices that we know about at this point in time are not widely used in the field (pharmacological treatments, motivational interviewing, cognitive behavioral, contingency management, and so on), whereas ineffective or potentially harmful approaches (confrontation, for example) are still widely used. The reasons for this lack of use of effective treatments and clinging to the old, less effective, or even harmful practices are numerous and complex. They are related to the lack of formal training of most substance abuse counselors, the fact that a significant portion of the workforce learned about treatment from their own treatment experiences or recovery process, and the lack of a universally accepted credentials or core competencies for substance abuse counselors. In addition, there is a dearth of education about substance abuse in the formal educational programs that train many future substance abuse professionals: medical schools, nursing schools, and social work and psychology programs. Even substance abuse counseling certificate programs inadequately address evidence-based practice. This must change.

The evidence-based practice movement is here to stay.

There are growing efforts at local, state, and federal agencies to define evidence-based practices and to incorporate research findings into practice. Thus far only one state, Oregon, has a mandate to demonstrate use of evidence-based practices, and it is too early to judge the success of that effort. The National Registry of Evidence-Based Programs and Practices (NREPP) is a federal effort to define and identify evidence-based practices for both the treatment and prevention fields. NREPP is still in its formative stages and offers little assistance to treatment providers at this point in time. Hopefully, it will be a good resource in the future. The evidence-based practice movement can be seen throughout the health and human services fields in the United States and Europe. The impetus to move research into practice is strong and growing.

There is a lack of guidance on implementation of evidence-based practices.

While the goal of infusing research into practice is noble and worthwhile, the means of accomplishing this task are not yet clear. There is a dearth of information about the best ways to implement evidence-based practices into field settings and measure their fidelity and impact on client outcomes. The Practice Improvement Collaborative network, funded by the Center for Substance Abuse Treatment (CSAT) from 1999 to 2004 was a good start, but more dedicated funding is needed to encourage research in this area because it is not often supported or rewarded by other research funding streams or by academic programs in universities.

There is a lack of incentives for forging research-practice collaborations.

Until the field increases the rewards for collaboration and decreases the negative consequences and barriers to collaboration, the movement will continue to proceed at a snail's pace. University department chairs and tenure and promotion committees often do not look favorably upon applied research, adoption studies, and time-consuming collaborative work with community agencies. Researchers need incentives to be involved in this important work. Policymakers and third-party payers do not generally require or provide incentives for agencies that partner with researchers or develop methods or resources for implementing evidence-based practices. Consequently, providers have little incentive or time to seek out these partnerships, and even if they are motivated to do so, there are no easy ways to find researchers who might match the needs of their agencies.

The field as a whole is not "research-savvy."

Providers have not been offered the skills that might help them to become more research-savvy consumers. More information about the research process in counselor credentialing and/or university educational programs would be helpful in many ways, from being able to understand and interpret research articles and reports, to grant-writing activities, to designing and carrying out program and intervention evaluations. Policymakers could also benefit from efforts to improve their research skills. Research process and methods need to be demystified.

Implications for the Field

All the evidence to date suggests that mandates to use evidence-based practices are premature, given the state of the art of treatment efficacy, effectiveness, and adoption and implementation studies. In spite of the significant limitations in the research base, there are movements in this direction of mandating use of evidence-based practices. The situation in Oregon will be of extreme interest to providers, researchers, and policymakers across the country. Will state mandates be the best method of infusing the field with research? Are providers equipped to be able to demonstrate use of evidence-based practices? Before mandating use of evidence-based practices, policymakers must consider what resources are needed for individual programs to identify and implement these practices. More money must be allocated to ongoing workgroups to identify effective practices; train and supervise staff in administering the practices; designing outcome and evaluation studies at the local, county, and state levels; measuring fidelity; and developing an infrastructure for monitoring whether programs actually follow through and use evidence-based practices. In addition, treatment providers and policymakers need to be given skills to be more research-savvy, and researchers need more experience and exposure to the real-world situations and priorities of the treatment delivery systems. These are preconditions for the evidence-based practice movement to succeed. An intermediate step between the current state of affairs and mandates to use evidence-based practice would be an incentive system that rewards agencies for taking steps toward more research-informed practices.

This book has focused on evidence-based practice, but there will always be a place for clinical guidelines, consensus documents, and practice improvement techniques. Manualized treatments will continue to be a good way of introducing more complex therapeutic approaches with the hope of greater fidelity, but will not be the sole answer. Improving substance abuse treatment will need to be multifaceted and include improving the education of substance abuse counselors, psychologists, nurses, physicians, and all helping professionals who work in the field, encouraging them to incorporate research-based practices at every level. Multi-pronged efforts that include evidence-based practices, clinical guidelines, practice improvements, and other tools are needed to really change the field. Complex problems demand comprehensive and broad-based solutions, not merely more treatment manuals.

Too much attention to only evidence-based, manualized treatments could result in neglect of the many other factors that influence treatment outcomes. Recall the four treatment factors of Hubble, Duncan, and Miller (1999): extratherapeutic factors, client-therapist relationship, hope/expectancy, and treatment approach. Evidence-based practices that attend to more than one of these factors are more likely to be effective. For example, motivational interviewing is an evidence-based practice that can be delivered via a manual, but it is also a therapeutic approach that helps improve the client-therapist relationship and may also increase the sense of hope and expectation of positive outcomes. On the other hand, rigid adherence to treatment manuals could negatively impact the client-therapist relationship and create a situation where clients do not feel they are getting individual attention from their counselors. There will always be a need to balance striving for fidelity with human qualities of spontaneity and genuineness.

Perhaps the most serious potential negative consequence of too hasty adoption of a rigid evidence-based practice model is the threat to cultural competency. The field has been challenged to consider issues of gender, ethnicity, immigrant status, sexuality, geographic region, religion and spirituality, age, and other individual differences that may impact access, retention, and response to treatment. Historically, substance abuse treatment practices were developed by and for middle-class men and have been applied, sometimes with modifications, to other groups. Many experts in the field have called for research on practices that were developed specifically on the theory and research of specific groups, such as Afrocentric practices, gender-responsive services, and urban youth programs (e.g., APA Presidential Task Force on Evidence-Based Practice, 2006; Castro & Garfinkle, 2003). The evidence base cannot be solely focused on "generic" treatments to be applied to all clients, but must stay attuned to the diversity of the treatment population, and of the staff who administer the treatments. Complex problems are rarely solved by generic, simple solutions.

Recommendations

The following recommendations are offered in the spirit of moving the field ahead, building stronger collaborations, and ultimately improving treatment service delivery and identifying the best therapeutic approaches with the best outcomes for clients. These recommendations could be considered as a form of strategic plan for the field as a whole.

1. Foster the development of research-practice collaborations.

- Funding sources will require or strongly recommend such collaborations in their calls for proposals. This may include research grant sources, such as the National Institutes of Health (NIH) and private foundations, as well as calls for service grants, such as CSAT and block grant monies.

- Academic departments will value and reward community outreach by faculty members and contribute to the development of "practice-based" research. Tenure and promotion decisions will be made on a balanced review of the value of research to communities served by universities, not just experimental rigor. Ultimately, researchers who partner with community agencies are better citizens.
- Journal editors will commit to publish the results of such collaborations, including articles about the implementation of evidence-based practice. More partnerships are forged between research and clinical journals and/or new journals are launched that are specifically devoted to translation of research into practice.
- Policymakers will reward such collaborations by offering incentives to agencies that seek out collaboration with researchers and/or infuse their agency with research-based practices.
- Academic training programs will make alterations in research training to better prepare researchers for community collaborations.
- Researchers will become regular speakers and presenters in counselor credentialing courses to begin to build common language and relationships.

2. *Continue the process of defining evidence-based practice.*
Groups will be formed to work collaboratively across disciplines to:

- Develop a common language.
- Establish criteria for evaluating evidence-based practices and set up a mechanism for ongoing updating of the research base, as well as evaluations of efforts to infuse research into practice.
- Keep criteria broad enough to encourage the development of new innovations, particularly in the area of cultural diversity.
- Balance empirical research on evidence-based practices with cultural competency, development of clinical skills and the therapeutic alliance, and attention to client needs.

3. *Identify mechanisms for enhancing the research skills of substance abuse treatment providers.*

- More research content will be added to the educational programs for counselors.
- Discussion of research will be infused into counselor credentialing programs to foster more positive attitudes about research.
- Continuing education courses (and incentives for taking them) will be developed.
- Educators who plan state and regional conferences for substance abuse treatment providers will screen presentations and workshops so that the focus is on evidence-based practices and research presentations that may inform practice.

4. Promote more extensive research on treatment effectiveness, implementation, and fidelity issues.

- Funding sources will commit funds specifically for such studies.
- More research-practice collaborations will be fostered through the existing Clinical Trials Network (keep it an open system rather than allowing it to become an insular group of select researchers and select providers).

5. Attention to cultural competency becomes a core value in the evidence-based practice movement.

- Research on evidence-based practices will consider issues of diversity at every level of the process, including members of diverse communities in the development of research questions, the development of treatment manuals or approaches, the recruitment and retention of participants, and the interpretation of results.
- Policymakers will construct broad definitions of evidence-based practice that allow for research on innovative new approaches and/or study of smaller subsets of the substance abusing population whose numbers can be obscured in large clinical trials.

Conclusions

In summary, the substance abuse treatment field is beginning to mature. A sign of this maturation is the growing pains experienced while trying to improve treatment outcomes. Research has begun to identify a number of factors that may improve outcomes; some of them are manualized therapy approaches, which are labeled as evidence-based practices in this book. However, evidence-based practices are only one of the many ways to improve substance abuse treatment. Hopefully, this book has provided a balanced account of evidence-based practices and interjected caution in the limitations of this approach. The development of research-practice partnerships may ultimately identify many other ways to improve services by use of research findings, and may find better ways to implement those manual-driven treatments. Given the nature of the problem of substance abuse, and the history of the treatment field, substance abuse treatment improvement will always be a complex matter, and the specific therapeutic practices or techniques just one small part of the puzzle. The work of identifying effective practices will be ongoing and never-ending, as advances in technology and understandings of substance abuse emerge, as patterns and types of substance use change, and as human conditions evolve. The evidence-based practice movement is one necessary step in the growth of the field, but as Miller, Zweben, and Johnson (2005) suggested:

Perhaps the proper attitude toward EBT [evidence-based treatment] is one of respect but not reverence. . . . There is danger that funders and regulators will take action prematurely, without good understanding of the state of the evidence and the practical constraints inherent in implementing worthy goals. A solid evidence base for the treatment services we provide is perhaps the best defense against extinction. (p. 274)

Glossary of Key Terms

Clinical practice guidelines: These are sets of statements or principles that are used to guide the clinical care of clients. Most specialty areas have clinical practice guidelines that were developed for and sponsored by professional associations. For example, the American Society of Addiction Medicine produces the guidelines for patient placement in substance abuse treatment.

Descriptive statistics: These statistical tools are used to characterize the sample or findings of a research study. They address questions such as: How many participants were there? How old were the participants? How many were women? What kinds of drug patterns were identified? What was the average score on a depression scale, and what was the range of scores? Common descriptive statistics include frequencies, percentages, ranges, means, and standard deviations.

Evidence-based practice (EBP): As used in this book, an EBP is a treatment approach or skill set that has been tested in several research studies, preferably with randomized clinical trials, and has found to be effective in impacting important client outcomes. It is in a form that is ready to implement in the field, such as a treatment manual or highly specific training materials.

Fidelity: This is the degree to which clinicians use an EBP in the same way that it was taught to them or presented in a manual.

Generalizability: The degree to which the findings of a research study might apply to clients or settings not included in the research study. To know if the findings of a study might generalize, one would need to look at the sample characteristics and how individuals were selected for the research study. If a program director is looking for an approach to use with women with anxiety disorders, but all the research on the approach has been done on antisocial men, the research may not generalize.

Hypothesis: Sometimes called a research question, the hypothesis sets out the expected outcome of the study ("Motivational interviewing will be better than treatment as usual in retaining adolescents in outpatient treatment") or specifies the question to be answered ("Does naltrexone reduce craving for gambling and tobacco along with reductions in craving for alcohol?").

Inferential statistics: These types of statistics are used to determine if the result of the study might be due to chance or sampling errors. They are used to compare the characteristics of a sample to the larger population to test representativeness, to compare the results from two groups to each other, or to compare some measure from baseline to posttest. Common inferential statistics include the t-test, ANOVA, chi square, and multiple regression analyses.

Logic model: An evaluation tool to facilitate program planning, intervention, and evaluation, a logic model is a visual way of showing the relationships among program resources, activities, and outcomes (results). These relationships can be depicted in tables, graphs, flow charts, or other forms. For a guide to developing logic models, see the W. K. Kellogg Foundation (2004): http://www.wkkf.org/default.aspx?tabid=101&CID=281&CatID=281&ItemID=2813669&NID=20&LanguageID=0

Meta-analysis: When several randomized clinical trials of one approach are available, those studies can be pooled together and studied for effect size. This method uses each study as the unit of analysis instead of pooling all the individual participants. Effect sizes can be nonexistent, small, medium, or large. Meta-analysis indicating medium or large effects is considered one of the strongest forms of scientific evidence for a practice.

p-value: Probability values indicate how likely that a result or outcome is due to chance or error. For exploratory studies, one might set the p-value fairly low, such as $p = 0.01$ (the chance of error is 1 in 100). For making decisions that involve risk or high cost, the p-value is often set at 0.001 (1 in 1,000 chance of being wrong).

Practice improvement: Also called process improvement, this includes strategies for enhancing the business components of a treatment delivery system, such as methods of reducing waiting lists, ways of handling drop-ins, altering program hours to accommodate more clients, and so on. The Network for the Improvement of Addiction Treatment (NIATx) provides many examples of these procedures. See http://chess.chsra.wisc.edu/NIATx/Content/Content Page.aspx?NID=171

Process evaluation: This procedure evaluates program characteristics, such as policies and procedures, rather than client outcomes. It is useful in the study of implementation of new approaches. Was the process—the way the approach was identified, the training, the adoption, the implementing procedures—effective? Process evaluation often uses methods such as interviews with staff members, focus groups, or review of meeting minutes as the primary data collection tools.

Randomized clinical trial (RCT): Often considered the gold standard of experimental studies used to determine the efficacy and/or effectiveness of some approach, an RCT has two components: random assignment of participants into groups; and at least two groups—an experimental and a control (no treatment) or comparison (treatment as usual) group.

Sample: In a research study, not everyone in the population of interest can be studied, so a sample of the population must be drawn. The population may be cocaine users, but the sample may be cocaine users in one urban clinic in an eastern state. Statistics can be used to determine if the sample is similar to the larger population on demographic characteristics, increasing the likelihood that the findings will generalize to the larger population.

Technology transfer: This term refers to the process of finding practical ways to apply scientific findings to the field. It includes tried and true methods such as workshop training, but broadens the idea to examine how and why people learn and how they can be taught or encouraged to apply the knowledge they are given consistently and maintain that knowledge base over time.

Treatment effectiveness: This term refers to whether an approach has demonstrated that it can produce positive results (impact a desired outcome) in a real-world treatment setting.

Treatment efficacy: This term refers to whether an approach has been demonstrated to work in controlled laboratory settings under ideal conditions.

Variable: A characteristic that can take on different values. Variables are the units of study in a research study. For example, gender is a variable that can take on the values of male, female, or other. Age is a variable that can take on many values, from 0 to 100 or more. In an experimental research study, there are at least two kinds of variables:

1. Dependent variables are the outcomes of interest (such as treatment completion rate).

2. Independent variables are the ones that the researcher manipulates (whether the client gets a contingency management intervention or treatment as usual).

References and Web Resources

References

Addiction Technology Transfer Center. (2000). *The change book.* Washington, DC: U.S. Department of Health and Human Services, Substance Abuse and Mental Health Services Administration, Center for Substance Abuse Treatment.

Addis, M. E. (1997). Evaluating the treatment manual as a means of disseminating empirically validated psychotherapies. *Clinical Psychology: Science and Practice, 4,* 1–11.

American Psychiatric Association. (1995). *Practice guidelines for the treatment of patients with substance use disorders: Alcohol, cocaine, opioids.* Washington, DC: Author.

American Society of Addiction Medicine. (2001). *Patient placement criteria for the treatment of substance-related disorders (PPC-2R).* Chevy Chase, MD: Author.

APA Presidential Task Force on Evidence-Based Practice. (2006). Evidence-based practice in psychology. *American Psychologist, 61*(4), 271–285.

Backer, T. (1993). Information alchemy: Transforming information through knowledge utilization. *Journal of the American Society for Information Science, 44*(4), 217–221.

Backer, T. (2003). Science-based strategic approaches to dissemination. In J. Sorensen, R. Rawson, J. Guydish, & J. Zweben (Eds.), *Drug abuse treatment through collaboration: Practice and research partnerships that work* (pp. 269–286). Washington, DC: American Psychological Association.

Balas, E., & Boren, S. (2000). Managing clinical knowledge for health care improvement. *Yearbook of Medical Informatics 2000.* Bethesda, MD: National Institute of Mental Health.

Ball, J. C., & Ross, A. (1991). *The effectiveness of methadone maintenance treatment.* New York: Springer-Verlag.

Ball, S., Bachrach, K., DeCarlo, J., Farentinos, C., Keen, M., McSherry, T., et al. (2002). Characteristics, beliefs, and practices of community clinicians trained to provide manual-guided therapy for substance abuse. *Journal of Substance Abuse Treatment, 23,* 309–318.

Barber, J., Luborsky, L., Crits-Chritoph, P., Thase, M., Weiss, R., Frank, A., et al. (1999). Therapeutic alliance as a predictor of outcome in treatment of cocaine dependence. *Psychotherapy Research, 9,* 54–73.

Barnett, P., & Hui, S. (2000). The cost-effectiveness of methadone maintenance. *The Mount Sinai Journal of Medicine, 67*(5/6), 365–374.

Batten, J., Horgan, C., Prottas, J., Simon, L., Larson, M., Elliott, E., et al. (1993). *Drug services research survey phase I final report: Non-correctional facilities.* Waltham, MA: Schneider Institutes for Health Policy, Brandeis University.

Bayer, A., Brisbane, F., & Ramirez, A. (1996). *Advanced methodological issues in culturally competent evaluation for substance abuse prevention* (Pub #SMA 96-3110). Rockville, MD: Department of Health and Human Services, Center for Substance Abuse Prevention.

Bell, D., Montoya, I., & Atkinson, J. (1997). Therapeutic connection and client progress in drug abuse treatment. *Journal of Clinical Psychology, 53*(3), 215–224.

Bellack, A. S., Bennett, M. E., Gearon, J. S., Brown, C. H., & Yang, Y. (2006). A randomized clinical trial of a new behavioral treatment for drug abuse in people with severe and persistent mental illness. *Archives of General Psychiatry, 63*(4), 426–432.

Beutler, L. (2004). The empirically supported treatments movement: A scientist-practitioner's response. *Clinical Psychology: Science and Practice, 11,* 225–229.

Blakely, C. H., Mayer, J. P., & Gottschalk, R. G. (1987). The fidelity-adaptation debate: Implications for the implementation of public sector social programs. *American Journal of Community Psychology, 15,* 253–268.

Bond, G. R. (2000). *Development of fidelity measures for psychiatric rehabilitation.* PRC Grantee Meeting, Washington, DC, October.

Bond, G. R., Evans, L., Salyers, M. P., Williams, J., & Kim, H. W. (2000). Measurement of fidelity in psychiatric rehabilitation. *Mental Health Services Research, 2*(2), 75–87.

Broner, N., Franczak, M., Dye, C., & McAllister, W. (2001). Knowledge transfer, policy-making, and community empowerment: A consensus model approach for providing public mental health and substance abuse services. *Psychiatric Quarterly, 72*(1), 79–102.

Burling, T., Marshall, G., & Seidner, A. (1991). Smoking cessation for substance abuse inpatients. *Journal of Substance Abuse, 3,* 264–276.

Califano, J. (2001). Preface. In National Center for Addiction and Substance Abuse, *Shoveling up: The impact of substance abuse on state budgets.* New York: Columbia University Press.

Carise, D., Cornely, W., & Gurel, O. (2002). A successful researcher-practitioner collaboration in substance abuse treatment. *Journal of Substance Abuse Treatment, 23,* 157–162.

Carroll, K. M. (1997). Manual-guided psychosocial treatment: A new virtual requirement for pharmacotherapy trials? *Archives of General Psychiatry, 54,* 923–928.

Carroll, K., Farentinos, C., Ball, S., Crits-Christoph, P., Libby, B., Morgenstern, J., et al. (2002). MET meets the real world: Design issues and clinical strategies in the Clinical Trials Network. *Journal of Substance Abuse Treatment, 23,* 73–80.

Castro, F. G., & Garfinkle, J. (2003). Critical issues in the development of culturally relevant substance abuse treatments for specific minority groups. *Alcoholism: Clinical and Experimental Research, 27,* 1381–1388.

Center for Substance Abuse Treatment. (1998). *Addiction counselor competencies: The knowledge, skills, and attitudes of professional practice.* Rockville, MD: U.S. Department of Health and Human Services, Substance Abuse and Mental Health Services Administration, Center for Substance Abuse Treatment.

Center for Substance Abuse Treatment. (1999). *Cultural issues in substance abuse treatment* (DHHS Pub. #SMA 99-3278). Rockville, MD: U.S. Department of Health and Human Services.

Center for Substance Abuse Treatment. (2000, November). *Changing the conversation: The National Treatment Plan Initiative.* Rockville, MD: U.S. Department of Health and Human Services, Substance Abuse and Mental Health Services Administration.

Centers for Disease Control and Prevention. (1999). Framework for program evaluation in public health. *MMWR, 48* (No. RR-11).

Craighead, W. E., & Craighead, L. W. (1998). Manual-based treatments: Suggestions for improving their clinical utility and acceptability. *Clinical Psychology: Science and Practice, 5,* 403–407.

Crits-Christoph, P., Frank, E., Chambless, D., Brody, C., & Karp, J. (1995). Training in empirically validated treatments: What are clinical psychology students learning? *Professional Psychology, Research and Practice, 26,* 514–522.

Davis, D., Thomson, M., Oxman, A., & Haynes, R. (1995). Changing physician performance: A systematic review of the effect of continuing education strategies. *Journal of the American Medical Association, 274,* 700–705.

Devine, P. (1999). *Using logic models in substance abuse treatment evaluations.* Rockville, MD: Substance Abuse and Mental Health Services Administration, Center for Substance Abuse Treatment.

Donovan, D. (2003). Relapse prevention in substance abuse treatment. In J. Sorensen, R. Rawson, J. Guydish, & J. Zweben (Eds.), *Drug abuse treatment through collaboration: Practice and research partnerships that work* (pp. 121–137). Washington, DC: American Psychological Association.

Dwyer, R., Richardson, D., Ross, M., Wodak, A., Miller, M., & Gold, J. (1994). A comparison of HIV risk between women and men who inject drugs. *AIDS Education and Prevention, 6,* 379–389.

Edmundson, E., Jr., & McCarty, D. (2005). *Implementing evidence-based practices for treatment of alcohol and drug disorders.* Binghamton, NY: Haworth.

Eldridge, G., St. Lawrence, J., Little, C., Shelby, M., Brasfield, T., Service, J., et al. (1997). Evaluation of an HIV risk reduction intervention for women entering inpatient substance abuse treatment. *AIDS Education and Prevention, 9*(Suppl. A), 62–76.

Eliason, M. J., & Amodia, D. S. (2006). A descriptive analysis of treatment outcomes for clients with co-occurring disorders: The role of minority identifications. *Journal of Dual Disorders, 2*(2), 89–109.

Eliason, M. J., Arndt, S., & Schut, A. (2006). Substance abuse counseling: What is treatment as usual? *Journal of Addictive Diseases, 24*(Suppl. 1), 33–52.

Fals-Stewart, W., & Birchler, G. (2001). A national survey of the use of couples therapy in substance abuse treatment. *Journal of Substance Abuse Treatment, 20,* 277–283.

Federal Register. (2006). DHSS, Notice regarding SAMHSA's NREPP: Priorities for NREPP reviews. Vol. 71 (126), 37590–37591.

Fetterman, D., & Wandersman, A. (Eds.). (2005). *Empowerment evaluation: Principles in practice.* New York: Guilford Press.

Finney, J. W., & Moos, R. H. (2002). Psychosocial treatments for alcohol use disorders. In P. Nathan & J. Gorman (Eds.), *A guide to treatments that work* (2nd ed., pp. 157–168). New York: Oxford University Press.

Friend, K. B., & Pagano, M. E. (2005). Smoking cessation and alcohol consumption in individuals in treatment for alcohol use disorders. *Journal of Addictive Disease, 24*(2), 61–75.

Gorski, T. (2000). CENAPS model of relapse prevention therapy. In J. Boren, L. Onken, & K. Carroll (Eds.), *Approaches to drug abuse counseling* (pp. 21–34). Bethesda, MD: National Institute on Drug Abuse.

Greco, P. J., & Eisenberg, J. M. (1993). Changing physician practices. *New England Journal of Medicine, 329,* 1271–1273.

Green, L. (2006). Public health asks of systems science: To advance our evidence-based practice, can you help us get more practice-based evidence? *American Journal of Public Health, 96*(3), 406–409.

Grella, C. (1999). Women in residential drug treatment: Differences by program type and pregnancy. *Journal of Health Care for the Poor and Underserved, 10,* 216–229.

Grella, C., Polinsky, M., Hser, Y., & Perry, S. (1999). Characteristics of women-only and mixed gender drug abuse treatment programs. *Journal of Substance Abuse Treatment, 17,* 37–44.

Guyatt, G., & Rennie, D. (2002). *Users' guide to the medical literature: A manual for evidence-based clinical practice.* Chicago: American Medical Association Press.

Hall, J. (1996). Pervasive effects of childhood sexual abuse in lesbians' recovery from alcohol problems. *Substance Use and Misuse, 31,* 225–239.

Havighurst, C., Hutt, P., McNeil, B., & Miller, W. (2001). Evidence: Its meaning in health care and law. *Journal of Health Politics, Policy, & Law, 26*(2), 195–215.

Hayes, S., Bissett, R., Roget, N., Padilla, M., Kohlenberg, B., Fisher, G., et al. (2004). The impact of acceptance and commitment training and multicultural training on the stigmatizing attitudes and professional burnout of substance abuse counselors. *Behavior Therapy, 35,* 821–835.

Higgins, S. T. (1996). Some potential contributions of reinforcement and consumer-demand theory to reducing cocaine use. *Addictive Behaviors, 21*(6), 803–816.

Higgins, S. T., Budney, A. J., Bickel, W. K., et al. (1993). Achieving cocaine abstinence with a behavioral approach. *American Journal of Psychiatry, 150,* 763–769.

Hilton, M. (2001). *Researcher in residence program: Experiences from New York State.* Rockville, MD: National Institute on Alcohol Abuse and Alcoholism.

Hubbard, R., Marsden, M., Rachal, J., Harwood, H. J., Cavanaugh, E. R., & Ginzburg, H. M. (1989). *Drug abuse treatment: A national study of effectiveness.* Chapel Hill: University of North Carolina Press.

Hubble, M., Duncan, B., & Miller, S. (1999). *The heart and soul of change: What works in therapy.* Washington, DC: American Psychological Association Press.

Humphreys, K., Wing, S., McCarty, D., Chappel, J., Gallant, L., Haberle, B., et al. (2004). Self-help organizations for alcohol and drug problems: Toward evidence-based practice and policy. *Journal of Substance Abuse Treatment, 26,* 151–158.

Institute of Behavioral Research, Texas Christian University. (2001/2002). DATAR-3: Building foundations for technology transfer. *Research Roundup, 11*(3/4), 1–6.

Institute of Medicine. (1990). *Treating drug problems, Vol. 1: A study of the evolution, effectiveness, and financing of public and private drug treatment systems.* Washington, DC: National Academy Press.

Institute of Medicine. (2001). *Crossing the quality chasm: A new health system for the 21st century.* Washington, DC: National Academy Press.

Jerrell, J. M., & Ridgely, M. S. (1999). Impact of robustness of program implementation on outcomes of clients in dual diagnosis programs. *Psychiatric Services, 50,* 109–112.

Jessup, M., Humphreys, J., Brindis, C., & Lee, K. (2003). Extrinsic barriers to substance abuse treatment among pregnant drug dependent women. *Journal of Drug Issues, 33*(2), 285–304.

Join Together. (2006). *A blueprint for the states: Policies to improve the ways states organize and deliver alcohol and drug prevention and treatment.* Boston: Join Together.

Joseph, A. M., Nichol, K. L., Willenbring, M., Korn, J. E., & Lysaght, L. S. (1990). Beneficial effects of treatment of nicotine dependence during an inpatient substance abuse treatment program. *Journal of the American Medical Association, 263,* 3043–3046.

Kalman, D., Hayes, K., Colby, S., Eaton, C., Rohsenow, D., & Monti, P. (2001). Concurrent versus delayed smoking cessation treatment for persons in early alcohol recovery: A pilot study. *Journal of Substance Abuse Treatment, 20,* 233–238.

Kasarabada, N., Hser, Y., Boles, S., & Huang, Y. (2002). Do patients' perceptions of their counselors influence outcomes of drug treatment? *Journal of Substance Abuse Treatment, 23,* 327–334.

Kaskutas, L. A., Greenfield, T. K., Borkman, T. J., & Room, J. A. (1998). Measuring treatment philosophy: A scale for substance abuse recovery programs. *Journal of Substance Abuse Treatment, 15,* 27–36.

Kiefer, F., & Mann, K. (2005). New achievements and pharmacotherapeutic approaches in the treatment of alcohol dependence. *European Journal of Pharmacology, 526,* 163–171.

Knight, J. (2004). A 35-year-old physician with opioid dependence. *Journal of the American Medical Association, 292*(11), 1351–1357.

Knight, K., Simpson, D., & Hiller, M. (1999). In-prison therapeutic communities in Texas: 3-year re-incarcerate outcomes. *The Prison Journal, 79*(3), 337–351.

Knudsen, H., & Roman, P. (2004). Modeling the use of innovations in private treatment organizations: The role of absorptive capacity. *Journal of Substance Abuse Treatment, 26,* 51–59.

Kranzler, H., & van Kirk, J. (2001). Efficacy of naltrexone and acamprosate for alcoholism treatments: A meta-analysis. *Alcoholism: Clinical and Experimental Research, 25,* 1335–1341.

Lamb, S., Greenlick, M., & McCarty, D. (1998). *Bridging the gap between practice and research: Forging partnerships with community-based drug and alcohol treatment.* Washington, DC: National Academy Press.

Lambert, M. (1992). Implications of outcome research for psychotherapy integration. In J. Norcross & M. Goldfried (Eds.), *Handbook of psychotherapy integration* (pp. 94–129). New York: Basic Books.

Leavitt, S. B. (2003). Evidence-based addiction medicine for practitioners: Evaluating and using research evidence in clinical practice. *Addiction Treatment Forum, March.* Retrieved December 8, 2006, from http://www.atforum.com/SiteRoot/pages/addiction_resources/EBAM_16_Pager.pdf

Lehman, W., Greener, J., & Simpson, D. (2002). Assessing organizational readiness for change. *Journal of Substance Abuse Treatment, 22,* 197–209.

Lemon, S. C., Friedmann, P. D., & Stein, M. D. (2003). The impact of smoking cessation on drug abuse treatment outcomes. *Addictive Behaviors, 28,* 1323–1331.

Linehan, M., Dimeff, L., Reynolds, S., Comtois, K., Shaw-Welch, S., Heagerty, P., et al. (2002). Dialectical behavior therapy versus comprehensive validation plus 12-step for the treatment of opioid-dependent women meeting criteria for borderline personality disorder. *Drug and Alcohol Dependence, 67,* 12–26.

Longshore, D., Grills, C., Anglin, M. D., & Annon, K. (1997). Desire for help among African American drug users. *Journal of Drug Users, 27,* 755–770.

Mark, T., Kranzler, H., Poole, V., Hagen, C. A., McLeod, C., & Crosse, S. (2003). Barriers to the use of medications to treat alcoholism. *American Journal on Addictions, 12,* 281–293.

Marlatt, G. A., & Gordon, J. (Eds.). (1985). *Relapse prevention.* New York: Guilford Press.

Marshall, P., Singer, M., & Clatts, M. (1999). *Integrating cultural observations and epidemiological approaches in the prevention of drug abuse and HIV/AIDS.* Rockville, MD: Department of Health and Human Services, National Institute on Drug Abuse.

Mattson, M. E., Del Boca, F. K., Carroll, K. M., Cooney, N. L., DiClemente, C. C., Donovan, D., et al. (1998). Compliance with treatment and follow-up protocols in project MATCH: Predictors and relationship to outcome. *Alcohol Clinical Experimental Research, 22*(6), 1328–1339.

McCarty, D., Rieckmann, T., Green, C., Gallon, S., & Knudsen, J. (2004). Training rural practitioners to use buprenorphine: Using the Change Book to facilitate technology transfer. *Journal of Substance Abuse Treatment, 26,* 203–208.

McCaughrin, W., & Howard, D. (1996). Variation in access to outpatient substance abuse treatment: Organizational factors and conceptual issues. *Journal of Substance Abuse, 8,* 403–415.

McCrady, B., & Ziedonis, D. (2001). American Psychiatric Association practice guidelines for substance use disorders. *Behavior Therapy, 32,* 309–336.

McDonnell, J., Nofs, D., & Hardman, M. (1989). An analysis of the procedural components of supported employment programs associated with employment outcomes. *Journal of Applied Behavior Analysis, 22,* 417–428.

McGovern, M., Fox, T., Xie, H., & Drake, R. (2004). A survey of clinical practices and readiness to adopt evidence-based practices: Dissemination research in an addiction treatment system. *Journal of Substance Abuse Treatment, 26,* 305–312.

McGraw, S. A., Sellers, D. E., Stone, E. J., Bebchuk, J., Edmundson, E. W., Johnson, C. C., et al. (1996). Using process data to explain outcomes: An illustration from the Child and Adolescent Trial for Cardiovascular Research. *Evaluation Review, 20*(3), 291–312.

McGrew, J. H., Bond, G. R., & Dietzen, L. L. (1994). Measuring the fidelity of implementation of a mental health program model. *Journal of Consulting and Clinical Psychology, 62,* 670–678.

McHugo, G. J., Drake, R. E., Teague, G. B., & Xie, H. (1999). Fidelity to assertive community treatment and client outcomes in the New Hampshire Dual Disorders Study. *Psychiatric Services, 50*(6), 818–824.

McLellan, A. T. (2006). Communicating across the "chasm": JSAT and Counselor initiate cooperative agreement. *Journal of Substance Abuse Treatment, 30*(1), 1.

McLellan, A. T., Lewis, D., O'Brien, C., & Kleber, H. (2000). Drug dependence: A chronic medical illness. *Journal of the American Medical Association, 284*(13), 1689–1695.

Meyer, R., & Mirin, S. (Eds.). (1979). *The heroin stimulus: Implications for a theory of addiction.* New York: Plenum.

Miller, M. (2006). The seductiveness of evidence. *Journal of Substance Abuse Treatment, 30,* 91–92.

Miller, S., Duncan, B., & Hubble, M. (2004). *Beyond integration: The triumph of outcome over process in clinical practice.* Chicago: Institute for the Study of Therapeutic Change.

Miller, W. R., & Brown, S. (1997). Why psychologists should treat alcohol and drug problems. *American Psychologist, 52,* 1269–1272.

Miller, W. R., & Rollnick, S. (2002). *Motivational interviewing: Helping people change.* New York: Guilford Press.

Miller, W. R., Sorensen, J., Selzer, J., & Brigham, G. (2006). Disseminating evidence-based practices in substance abuse treatment: A review with suggestions. *Journal of Substance Abuse Treatment, 31,* 25–39.

Miller, W. R., & Wilbourne, P. (2002). Mesa Grande: A methodological analysis of clinical trials of treatments for alcohol use disorders. *Addiction, 97,* 265–277.

Miller, W. R., Wilbourne, P., & Hettema, J. (2003). What works? A summary of alcohol treatment outcome research. In R. Hester & W. R. Miller (Eds.), *Handbook of alcoholism treatment approaches: Effective alternatives* (3rd ed., pp. 13–63). Boston: Allyn & Bacon.

Miller, W. R., Yahne, C., Moyers, T., Martinez, J., & Perritano, M. (2004). A randomized trial of methods to help clinicians learn motivational interviewing. *Journal of Consulting and Clinical Psychology, 72,* 1050–1062.

Miller, W. R., Zweben, J., & Johnson, W. (2005). Evidence-based treatment: Why, what, where, when, and how? *Journal of Substance Abuse Treatment, 29*(4), 267–276.

Morgenstern, J. (2000). Effective technology transfer in alcoholism treatment. *Substance Use and Misuse, 35,* 1659–1678.

Morgenstern, J., Morgan, T., McCrady, B., Keller, D., & Carroll, K. (2001). Manual-guided cognitive-behavioral therapy training: A promising method for disseminating empirically supported substance abuse treatments to the practice community. *Psychology of Addictive Behaviors, 15,* 83–88.

Mulligan, D., McCarty, D., Potter, D., & Krakow, M. (1985). Counselors in public and private alcoholism and drug abuse treatment programs. *Alcoholism Treatment Quarterly, 6*(3/4), 75–89.

Najavits, L. (2002). *Seeking safety: A treatment manual for PTSD and substance abuse.* New York: Guilford Press.

National Center for Addiction and Substance Abuse. (2001). *Shoveling up: The impact of substance abuse on state budgets.* New York: Columbia University Press.

National Institute on Drug Abuse. (1999). *Principles of drug addiction treatment: A research-based guide* (NIH Publication No. 99-4180). Bethesda, MD: National Institutes of Health.

National Institutes of Health. (1997, November). *NIH consensus development statement on effective medical treatment of heroin addiction, 15*(6), 15–19.

O'Brien, C. P., & McKey, J. (2002). Pharmacological treatments for substance use disorders. In P. Nathan & J. Gorman (Eds.), *A guide to treatments that work* (2nd ed., pp. 125–156). New York: Oxford University Press.

O'Connor, P., Oliveto, A., Shi, J., Triffleman, E. G., Carroll, K. M., Kosten, T. R., et al. (1998). A randomized trial of buprenorphine maintenance for heroin dependence in a primary care clinic for substance users versus a methadone clinic. *American Journal of Medicine, 105,* 100–105.

O'Malley, S. (1998). *Naltrexone and alcoholism treatment* (CSAT TIP Series 28, Pub #SMA-90-3206). Rockville, MD: Substance Abuse and Mental Health Services Administration.

Oregon Office of Mental Health and Addiction Services. (2006). *Progress report on the implementation of evidence-based practices* (draft). Salem: Oregon Department of Human Services. Retrieved May 2, 2006, from http://egov.oregon.gov/DHS/mentalhealth/ebp/main.shtml

Orwin, R. G. (2000). Assessing program fidelity in substance abuse health services research. *Addiction, 95*(Suppl. 3), S309–S327.

Orwin, R. G., Francisco, L., & Bernichon, J. (2001). *Effectiveness of women's substance abuse treatment programs: A meta-analysis.* Arlington, VA: Substance Abuse and Mental Health Services Administration, Center for Substance Abuse Treatment.

Owen, P. (2003). *Measuring treatment progress: An outcome study guidebook.* Center City, MN: Hazelden Press.

Paul, J., Barnett, D., Crosby, M., & Stall, R. (1996). Longitudinal changes in alcohol and drug use among men seen at a gay-specific substance abuse treatment agency. *Journal of Studies on Alcohol, 57,* 475–485.

Peters, R., Moore, K., Hills, H., Young, M. S., LeVasseur, J., Rich, A., et al. (2005). Use of opinion leaders and intensive training to implement evidence-based co-occurring disorders treatment in the community. In E. Edmundson, Jr., & D. McCarty (Eds.), *Implementing evidence-based practices for treatment of alcohol and drug disorders* (pp. 53–74). Binghamton, NY: Haworth.

Project Match Research Group. (1998). Therapist effects in three treatments for alcohol problems. *Psychotherapy Research, 8,* 455–474.

Rawson, R., Marinelli-Casey, P., & Ling, W. (2002). Dancing with strangers: Will U.S. substance abuse practice and research organizations build mutually productive relationships? *Addictive Behaviors, 27,* 941–949.

Richter, K., Ahluwalia, H., Mosier, M., Nazir, N., & Ahluwalia, J. S. (2002). A population-based study of cigarette smoking among illicit drug users in the United States. *Addiction, 97,* 861–869.

Rogers, E. (1995). *The diffusion of innovations* (4th ed.). New York: The Free Press.

Roman, P., & Johnson, J. (2002). Adoption and implementation of new technologies in substance abuse treatment. *Journal of Substance Abuse Treatment, 22,* 211–218.

Roman, P., Johnson, J., & Blum, T. (2000). The transformation of private substance abuse treatment: The results of a national study. In J. Levy (Ed.), *Advances in medical sociology* (Vol. 7, pp. 321–342). Greenwich, CT: JAI Press.

Ross, H., Swinson, R., Doumani, S., & Larkin, E. (1995). Diagnosing co-morbidity in substance abusers: A comparison of the test-retest reliability of two interviews. *American Journal of Drug and Alcohol Abuse, 21,* 167–185.

Sackett, D., Rosenberg, W., Gray, J., Haynes, R., & Richardson, W. (1996). Evidence-based medicine: What it is and what it isn't. *British Medical Journal, 312,* 71–72.

Schultz, S. K., Arndt, S., & Liesveld, J. (2003). Locations of facilities with special programs for older substance abuse clients in the U.S. *Journal of the American Geriatric Association, 18*(9), 839–843.

Schutte, K., Nichols, K., Brennan, P., & Moos, R. (2003). A ten-year follow-up of older former drinkers: Risk of relapse and implications of successfully sustained remission. *Journal of Studies on Alcohol, 64*(3), 367–374.

Scott, C. K., Ross, M. A., & Dennis, M. I. (2004). Pathways in the relapse-treatment-recovery cycle over three years. *Journal of Substance Abuse Treatment, 28*(1) (Suppl. 1), S63–S72.

Sechrest, L., Backer, T., Rogers, E., Campbell, T., & Grady, M. (Eds.). (1994). *Effective dissemination of clinical and health information.* Rockville, MD: Agency for Health Care Policy and Research.

Sholomskas, D., Syracuse-Siewert, G., Rounsaville, B., Ball, S., Nuro, K., & Carroll, K. (2005). We don't train in vain: A dissemination trail of three strategies of training clinicians in cognitive-behavioral therapy. *Journal of Consulting and Clinical Psychology, 73,* 106–115.

Shoptaw, S., Rotheram-Fuller, E., Yang, X., Frosch, D., Nahom, D., Jarvik, M., et al. (2002). Smoking cessation in methadone maintenance. *Addiction, 97,* 1317–1328.

Simpson, D. (2002). A conceptual framework for transferring research to practice. *Journal of Substance Abuse Treatment, 22,* 171–182.

Simpson, D., & Brown, B. (1999). Special issue: Treatment process and outcome studies from DATOS. *Drug and Alcohol Dependence, 57*(2), 81–174.

Sorensen, J., Hall, S., Loeb, P., Allen, T., Glaser, E., & Greenberg, P. (1988). Dissemination of a job seekers' workshop to a drug treatment program. *Behavior Therapy, 19,* 143–155.

Sorensen, J., Rawson, R., Guydish, J., & Zweben, J. (Eds.). (2003). *Drug abuse treatment through collaboration: Practice and research partnerships that work.* Washington, DC: American Psychological Association.

Streeton, C., & Whelan, G. (2001). Naltrexone, a relapse prevention maintenance treatment of alcohol dependence: A meta-analysis of randomized controlled trials. *Alcohol and Alcoholism, 36,* 544–552.

Taylor, V. (1993). *Women drug users.* Oxford, UK: Clarendon Press.

Teague, G. B., Drake, B., & Ackerman, T. (1995). Evaluating use of continuous treatment teams for persons with mental illness and substance abuse. *Psychiatric Services, 46,* 689–695.

Thomas, V., Melchert, T., & Banker, J. (1999). Substance dependence and personality disorders: Co-morbidity and treatment outcomes in an inpatient treatment population. *Journal of Studies on Alcohol, 60,* 271–277.

Tucker, J., & Roth, D. (2006). Extending the evidence hierarchy to enhance evidence-based practice for substance use disorders. *Addiction, 101,* 918–932.

United Way of America. (1996). *Measuring program outcomes: A practical approach.* Alexandria, VA: Author.

Valente, T. (2002). *Evaluating health promotion programs.* New York: Oxford University Press.

Victora, C., Habicht, J., & Bryce, J. (2004). Evidence-based public health: Moving beyond randomized trials. *American Journal of Public Health, 94*(3), 400–405.

White, W. (1998). *Slaying the dragon: The history of addiction treatment and recovery in America.* Bloomington, IL: Chestnut Health Systems.

Web Resources

Addiction Technology Transfer Center (ATTC) national Web site: www.nattc.org

American Society of Addiction Medicine (ASAM) Web site: www.asam.org

Center for Alcohol and Substance Abuse at Columbia University Web site: http://www.casacolumbia.org/

Center for Substance Abuse Research (CESAR) Web site: http://www.cesar.umd.edu/

Institute for Behavioral Research, Texas Christian University Web site: http://www.ibr.tcu.edu/

Join Together Web site: www.jointogether.org

National Registry for Evidence-Based Practices and Programs (NREPP) Web site: http://modelprograms.samhsa.gov/template.cfm?page=nreppover

Practice Improvement Collaborative (PIC) national Web site: www.samhsa.gov/centers/csat/content/pic

Robert Wood Johnson Foundation (RWJF) Paths to Recovery Web site: www.niatx.org

Appendix A

Text of Oregon Law

72nd OREGON LEGISLATIVE ASSEMBLY—2003 Regular Session

Enrolled Senate Bill 267

Sponsored by COMMITTEE ON JUDICIARY (at the request of AFSCME Council 75)

CHAPTER ....

AN ACT

Relating to public safety; creating new provisions; amending ORS 181.620 and 181.637; and declaring an emergency.

Be It Enacted by the People of the State of Oregon:

SECTION 1. ORS 181.620 is amended to read:

181.620. (1) The Governor shall appoint a Board on Public Safety Standards and Training consisting of [23] 24 members as follows:
  (a) Two members shall be chiefs of police recommended to the Governor by the Oregon Association of Chiefs of Police;
  (b) One member shall be a sheriff recommended to the Governor by the Oregon State Sheriffs' Association;
  (c) One member shall be a fire chief recommended to the Governor by the Oregon Fire Chiefs' Association;

(d) One member shall be a representative of the fire service recommended to the Governor by the Oregon Fire District Directors' Association;

(e) One member shall be a member of the Oregon State Fire Fighter's Council recommended to the Governor by the executive body of the council;

(f) One member shall be a representative of corrections personnel recommended to the Governor by the Oregon State Sheriffs' Association;

(g) One member shall be a representative of the fire service recommended to the Governor by the Oregon Volunteer Fire Fighters' Association;

(h) One member shall be a representative of public safety telecommunicators;

(i) One member shall be a district attorney recommended to the Governor by the Oregon District Attorneys Association;

(j) One member shall be the Superintendent of State Police;

(k) One member shall be the Chief of the Portland Police Bureau;

(l) One member shall be the State Fire Marshal;

(m) One member shall be the Chief of the Portland Fire Bureau;

(n) One member shall be the Director of the Department of Corrections;

(o) One member shall be the Special Agent in Charge of the Federal Bureau of Investigation for Oregon;

(p) One member shall represent forest protection agencies recommended to the Governor by the State Forestry Department;

(q) One member shall be an administrator of a municipality recommended to the Governor by the executive body of the League of Oregon Cities;

(r) Two members shall be nonmanagement representatives of law enforcement;

(s) One member shall be a public member. A person appointed as a public member under this section shall be a person:
     (A) Who has no personal interest or occupational responsibilities in the area of responsibility given to the board; and
     (B) Who represents the interests of the public in general; [and]

(t) Two members shall be representatives of the private security industry recommended to the Governor by the Advisory Committee on Private Security Services; and

(u) One member shall be a representative of the collective bargaining unit that represents the largest number of individual workers in the Department of Corrections.

(2) The term of office of a member is three years, and no member may be removed from office except for cause. Before the expiration of the term of a member, the Governor shall appoint the member's successor to assume the member's duties on July 1 next following. In case of a vacancy for any cause, the Governor shall make an appointment, effective immediately, for the unexpired term.

(3) Except for members who serve by virtue of office, no member shall serve more than two terms. For purposes of this subsection, a person appointed to fill a vacancy consisting of an unexpired term of at least one and one-half years has served a full term.

(4) Appointments of members of the board by the Governor, except for those members who serve by virtue of office, are subject to confirmation by the Senate in the manner provided in ORS 171.562 and 171.565.

(5) A member of the board is entitled to compensation and expenses as provided in ORS 292.495.

SECTION 2. ORS 181.637 is amended to read:

181.637. (1) The Board on Public Safety Standards and Training shall establish the following policy committees:
    (a) Corrections Policy Committee;
    (b) Fire Policy Committee;
    (c) Police Policy Committee; and
    (d) Telecommunications Policy Committee.

(2) The members of each policy committee shall select a chairperson and vice chairperson for the policy committee. Only members of the policy committee who are also members of the board are eligible to serve as a chairperson or vice chairperson. The vice chairperson may act as chairperson in the absence of the chairperson.

(3) The Corrections Policy Committee consists of:
    (a) All of the board members who represent the corrections discipline;
    (b) The chief administrative officer of the training division of the Department of Corrections;
    (c) A security manager from the Department of Corrections; and
    (d) The following, who may not be current board members, appointed by the chairperson of the board:
        (A) One person recommended by and representing the Oregon State Sheriffs' Association;

    (B) Two persons recommended by and representing the Oregon Jail Managers' Association;

    (C) One person recommended by and representing a statewide association of community corrections directors; [and]

    (D) One nonmanagement corrections officer employed by the Department of Corrections; and

    (E) One corrections officer who is a female, who is employed by the Department of Corrections at a women's correctional facility and who is a member of a bargaining unit.

(4) The Fire Policy Committee consists of:

  (a) All of the board members who represent the fire service discipline; and

  (b) The following, who may not be current board members, appointed by the chairperson of the board:

    (A) One person recommended by and representing a statewide association of fire instructors;

    (B) One person recommended by and representing a statewide association of fire marshals;

    (C) One person recommended by and representing community college fire programs; and

    (D) One nonmanagement firefighter recommended by a statewide organization of firefighters.

(5) The Police Policy Committee consists of:

  (a) All of the board members who represent the law enforcement discipline; and

  (b) The following, who may not be current board members, appointed by the chairperson of the board:

    (A) One person recommended by and representing the Oregon Association of Chiefs of Police;

    (B) Two persons recommended by and representing the Oregon State Sheriffs' Association;

    (C) One command officer recommended by and representing the Oregon State Police; and

    (D) One nonmanagement law enforcement officer.

(6) The Telecommunications Policy Committee consists of:

  (a) All of the board members who represent the telecommunications discipline; and

  (b) The following, who may not be current board members, appointed by the chairperson of the board:

(A) Two persons recommended by and representing a statewide association of public safety communications officers;

(B) One person recommended by and representing the Oregon Association of Chiefs of Police;

(C) One person recommended by and representing the Oregon State Police;

(D) Two persons representing telecommunicators;

(E) One person recommended by and representing the Oregon State Sheriffs' Association;

(F) One person recommended by and representing the Oregon Fire Chiefs' Association;

(G) One person recommended by and representing the Emergency Medical Services and Trauma Systems Program of the Department of Human Services; and

(H) One person representing paramedics and recommended by a statewide association dealing with fire medical issues.

(7) In making appointments to the policy committees under this section, the chairperson of the board shall seek to reflect the diversity of the state's population. An appointment made by the chairperson of the board must be ratified by the board before the appointment is effective. The chairperson of the board may remove an appointed member for just cause. An appointment to a policy committee that is based on the member's employment is automatically revoked if the member changes employment. The chairperson of the board shall fill a vacancy in the same manner as making an initial appointment. The term of an appointed member is two years. An appointed member may be appointed to a second term.

(8) A policy committee may meet at such times and places as determined by the policy committee in consultation with the board. A majority of a policy committee constitutes a quorum to conduct business. A policy committee may create subcommittees if needed.

(9)(a) Each policy committee shall develop policies, requirements, standards and rules relating to its specific discipline. A policy committee shall submit its policies, requirements, standards and rules to the board for the board's consideration. When a policy committee submits a policy, requirement, standard or rule to the board for the board's consideration, the board shall:

(A) Approve the policy, requirement, standard or rule;

(B) Disapprove the policy, requirement, standard or rule; or

(C) Defer a decision and return the matter to the policy committee for revision or reconsideration.

(b) The board may defer a decision and return a matter submitted by a policy committee under paragraph (a) of this subsection only once. If a policy, requirement, standard or rule that was returned to a policy committee is resubmitted to the board, the board shall take all actions necessary to implement the policy, requirement, standard or rule unless the board disapproves the policy, requirement, standard or rule.

(c) Disapproval of a policy, requirement, standard or rule under paragraph (a) or (b) of this subsection requires a two-thirds vote by the members of the board.

(10) At any time after submitting a matter to the board, the chairperson of the policy committee may withdraw the matter from the board's consideration.

SECTION 3. As used in this section and section 7 of this 2003 Act:

(1) "Agency" means:
    (a) The Department of Corrections;
    (b) The Oregon Youth Authority;
    (c) The State Commission on Children and Families;
    (d) That part of the Department of Human Services that deals with mental health and addiction issues; and
    (e) The Oregon Criminal Justice Commission.

(2) "Cost effective" means that cost savings realized over a reasonable period of time are greater than costs.

(3) "Evidence-based program" means a program that:
    (a) Incorporates significant and relevant practices based on scientifically based research; and
    (b) Is cost effective.

(4)(a) "Program" means a treatment or intervention program or service that is intended to:
    (A) Reduce the propensity of a person to commit crimes;
    (B) Improve the mental health of a person with the result of reducing the likelihood that the person will commit a crime or need emergency mental health services; or
    (C) Reduce the propensity of a person who is less than 18 years of age to engage in antisocial behavior with the result of reducing the likelihood that the person will become a juvenile offender.

(b) "Program" does not include:

    (A) An educational program or service that an agency is required to provide to meet educational requirements imposed by state law; or

    (B) A program that provides basic medical services.

(5) "Scientifically based research" means research that obtains reliable and valid knowledge by:

    (a) Employing systematic, empirical methods that draw on observation or experiment;

    (b) Involving rigorous data analyses that are adequate to test the stated hypotheses and justify the general conclusions drawn; and

    (c) Relying on measurements or observational methods that provide reliable and valid data across evaluators and observers, across multiple measurements and observations and across studies by the same or different investigators.

SECTION 4. As used in sections 5 and 6 of this 2003 Act, "agency," "cost effective," "evidence-based program" and "program" have the meanings given those terms in section 3 of this 2003 Act.

SECTION 5. (1) For the biennium beginning July 1, 2005, the Department of Corrections, the Oregon Youth Authority, the State Commission on Children and Families, that part of the Department of Human Services that deals with mental health and addiction issues and the Oregon Criminal Justice Commission shall spend at least 25 percent of state moneys that each agency receives for programs on evidence-based programs.

(2) Each agency shall submit a report containing:

    (a) An assessment of each program on which the agency expends funds, including but not limited to whether the program is an evidence-based program;

    (b) The percentage of state moneys the agency receives for programs that is being expended on evidence-based programs;

    (c) The percentage of federal and other moneys the agency receives for programs that is being expended on evidence-based programs; and

    (d) A description of the efforts the agency is making to meet the requirements of subsection (1) of this section and sections 6 (1) and 7 (1) of this 2003 Act.

(3) The agencies shall submit the reports required by subsection (2) of this section no later than September 30, 2006, to the interim legislative committee dealing with judicial matters.

(4) If an agency, during the biennium beginning July 1, 2005, spends more than 75 percent of the state moneys that the agency receives for programs on programs that are not evidence based, the Legislative Assembly shall consider the agency's failure to meet the requirement of subsection (1) of this section in making appropriations to the agency for the following biennium.

(5) Each agency may adopt rules necessary to carry out the provisions of this section, including but not limited to rules defining a reasonable period of time for purposes of determining cost effectiveness.

SECTION 6. (1) For the biennium beginning July 1, 2007, the Department of Corrections, the Oregon Youth Authority, the State Commission on Children and Families, that part of the Department of Human Services that deals with mental health and addiction issues and the Oregon Criminal Justice Commission shall spend at least 50 percent of state moneys that each agency receives for programs on evidence-based programs.

(2) Each agency shall submit a report containing:
  (a) An assessment of each program on which the agency expends funds, including but not limited to whether the program is an evidence-based program;
  (b) The percentage of state moneys the agency receives for programs that is being expended on evidence-based programs;
  (c) The percentage of federal and other moneys the agency receives for programs that is being expended on evidence-based programs; and
  (d) A description of the efforts the agency is making to meet the requirements of subsection (1) of this section and section 7 (1) of this 2003 Act.

(3) The agencies shall submit the reports required by subsection (2) of this section no later than September 30, 2008, to the interim legislative committee dealing with judicial matters.

(4) If an agency, during the biennium beginning July 1, 2007, spends more than 50 percent of the state moneys that the agency receives for programs on programs that are not evidence based, the Legislative Assembly shall consider the agency's failure to meet the requirement of subsection (1) of this section in making appropriations to the agency for the following biennium.

(5) Each agency may adopt rules necessary to carry out the provisions of this section, including but not limited to rules defining a reasonable period of time for purposes of determining cost effectiveness.

SECTION 7. (1) The Department of Corrections, the Oregon Youth Authority, the State Commission on Children and Families, that part of the Department of Human Services that deals with mental health and addiction issues and the Oregon Criminal Justice Commission shall spend at least 75 percent of state moneys that each agency receives for programs on evidence-based programs.

(2) Each agency shall submit a biennial report containing:
  (a) An assessment of each program on which the agency expends funds, including but not limited to whether the program is an evidence-based program;
  (b) The percentage of state moneys the agency receives for programs that is being expended on evidence-based programs;
  (c) The percentage of federal and other moneys the agency receives for programs that is being expended on evidence-based programs; and
  (d) A description of the efforts the agency is making to meet the requirement of subsection (1) of this section.

(3) The agencies shall submit the reports required by subsection (2) of this section no later than September 30 of each even-numbered year to the interim legislative committee dealing with judicial matters.

(4) If an agency, in any biennium, spends more than 25 percent of the state moneys that the agency receives for programs on programs that are not evidence based, the Legislative Assembly shall consider the agency's failure to meet the requirement of subsection (1) of this section in making appropriations to the agency for the following biennium.

(5) Each agency may adopt rules necessary to carry out the provisions of this section, including but not limited to rules defining a reasonable period of time for purposes of determining cost effectiveness.

SECTION 8. The provisions of section 7 of this 2003 Act apply to biennia beginning on or after July 1, 2009.

SECTION 9. (1) As used in this section, "agency," "evidence-based program" and "program" have the meanings given those terms in section 3 of this 2003 Act.

(2) Each agency shall conduct an assessment of existing programs and establish goals that enable the agency to meet the requirements of sections 5 (1), 6 (1) and 7 (1) of this 2003 Act. Each agency shall work with interested persons to establish the goals and to develop a process for meeting the goals.

(3) No later than September 30, 2004, each agency shall submit a report containing:

    (a) An assessment of each program on which the agency expends funds, including but not limited to whether the program is an evidence-based program;

    (b) The percentage of state moneys the agency receives for programs that is being expended on evidence-based programs;

    (c) The percentage of federal and other moneys the agency receives for programs that is being expended on evidence-based programs; and

    (d) A description of the efforts the agency is making to meet the requirements of sections 5 (1), 6 (1) and 7 (1) of this 2003 Act.

SECTION 10. This 2003 Act being necessary for the immediate preservation of the public peace, health and safety, an emergency is declared to exist, and this 2003 Act takes effect on its passage.

Passed by Senate March 5, 2003

Repassed by Senate July 24, 2003

....

Secretary of Senate

....

President of Senate

Passed by House June 24, 2003

Repassed by House July 29, 2003

....

Speaker of House

Received by Governor:

.........................M.,.., 2003

Approved:

........................M.,.., 2003

....
Governor

Filed in Office of Secretary of State:

........................M.,.., 2003

....
Secretary of State

Index

177

About the Author

Michele (Mickey) J. Eliason, PhD, is an adjunct professor at the Institute for Health and Aging at the University of California, San Francisco. She also teaches courses about sexuality and gender at San Francisco State University. Formerly, she was a faculty member in the College of Nursing at the University of Iowa for nearly 20 years. Dr. Eliason has been an applied researcher in the substance abuse treatment field for more than 15 years, and is particularly interested in diverse populations, including women and sexual and gender minority clients. Her interest in the evidence-based practice movement grew out of a 4-year involvement with the Iowa Practice Improvement Collaborative, funded by the Center for Substance Abuse Treatment to develop a statewide practice-research collaboration. This highly rewarding experience highlighted the complex barriers to implementing evidence-based practices in the poorly funded and stigmatized settings of community-based treatment programs.